LEAN
DONE RIGHT

LEAN
DONE RIGHT

ACHIEVE AND MAINTAIN REFORM
IN YOUR **HEALTHCARE ORGANIZATION**

Thomas G. Zidel

ACHE Management Series

Library of Congress Cataloging-in-Publication Data

Zidel, Tom, 1949-
   Lean done right : achieve and maintain reform in your healthcare organization / Thomas G. Zidel.
      p. cm.
   Includes bibliographical references and index.
   ISBN 978-1-56793-422-9 (alk. paper)
 1. Health services administration. 2. Industrial efficiency. 3. Lean manufacturing. I. Title.
   RA971.Z528 2012
   362.1068--dc23

                                        2011046403

The paper used in this publication meets the minimum requirements of American National Standard for Information Sciences—Permanence of Paper for Printed Library Materials, ANSI Z39.48-1984. ∞™

Acquisitions editor: Janet Davis; Project manager: Jennifer Seibert; Cover designer: Marisa Jackson; Layout: Scott Miller

Found an error or a typo? We want to know! Please e-mail it to hap1@ache.org, and put "Book Error" in the subject line.

For photocopying and copyright information, please contact Copyright Clearance Center at www.copyright.com or at (978) 750–8400.

Health Administration Press
A division of the Foundation of the American
    College of Healthcare Executives
One North Franklin Street, Suite 1700
Chicago, IL 60606–3529
(312) 424–2800

To Liz, Sam, Betsy, and Brooke

Contents

Preface

In 1985 the three senior managers of the International Motor Vehicle Program at the Massachusetts Institute of Technology—Daniel Roos, Daniel Jones, and James Womack—traveled to Japan to conduct a detailed study of Toyota's manufacturing methods. Five years later they published the results of this study in a book titled *The Machine That Changed the World*. This book compared the mass production methods used throughout the world to the Toyota Production System and introduced North American and Western European manufacturing companies to the concept of Lean.

The book quickly became a best seller in the US manufacturing industry, and many American companies attempted to adopt Lean methods. These manufacturing companies wanted to experience the benefits that Lean had to offer, but on their own terms. They wanted to produce more, pay less, and eliminate problems, but they did not necessarily want to change or were incapable of changing. They attempted to superimpose Lean methods on their existing mass production processes and disregarded many Lean principles, such as improved communication, empowerment, and teamwork. They viewed Lean simply as a set of problem-solving tools, and the vehicle for Lean implementation was the kaizen event.

During my 20 years working in manufacturing, I have seen many organizations attempt to become Lean. Some of these organizations were successful. Many more were not. The difference between these organizations was not the product they produced or the service they provided. Their success did not depend on union involvement or the complexity of their existing processes. The difference was their approach to Lean implementation. Organizations that took the approach described in the previous paragraph seldom were successful. Those that succeeded took the time to create a culture of continuous improvement, fostered systems thinking, and deployed Lean tools and principles strategically.

The ineffective approach to Lean seen in the manufacturing industry permeates many healthcare organizations today and is a direct route to failure. This book provides a road map for proper Lean implementation that will lead to real healthcare reform. The model introduced in this book discourages organizations from using Lean tools simply to address problem areas and focuses on strategically directed action, developing a Lean organizational culture, and enhancing the care delivery system.

The first section of the book expounds on the problems with existing implementation strategies, introduces the culture-based implementation model, and highlights the need for strategic direction. The second section dissects the culture-creating path into steps, explains the rationale for each step, and lays out the order in which the steps should be implemented. The third section does the same for the system-creating path.

Hospitals and other healthcare organizations cannot afford to waste time, money, and resources on improper Lean implementation. They must get it right the first time. Many organizations employ outside consultants to launch a Lean initiative, only to have the effort fall apart when the consultants depart. The model described in this book will put your organization on the road to success and enable it to sustain the Lean initiative independently.

The journey through this model is neither quick nor easy, but for organizations willing to make the commitment and follow the model diligently, it is an exciting and rewarding experience.

Thomas G. Zidel

Introduction

President Barack Obama identified healthcare costs as "one of the greatest threats, not just to the well-being of our families and the prosperity of our businesses, but to the very foundation of our economy" (White House Forum on Health Reform 2009). The increasing cost of healthcare is possibly the greatest financial crisis facing our nation today. Nightly news broadcasts report statistically significant data related to cost overruns of billions of dollars and a national debt of trillions of dollars. This constant barrage of financial facts has rendered us immune to the shock these numbers should produce.

Even more disturbing is that much of the cost of healthcare is the result of waste and is manifested as errors, unnecessary testing, inefficiencies, and more. Studies have estimated that 30 to 40 cents of every dollar spent in healthcare is the result of waste (National Coalition on Health Care 2009). Moreover, the quality of healthcare has diminished significantly. Patients are injured; improperly medicated; infected; and exposed to unnecessary, anxiety-producing, and sometimes painful tests. Some patients die—the ultimate cost of poor quality in healthcare.

Bailouts are not the solution to these problems, and dialogue with insurance companies, pharmaceutical companies, or medical equipment manufacturers won't change the situation. Likewise, socialized medicine would generate more waste; fewer healthcare providers would be attempting to care for a growing population that is living longer than ever before in history. These strategies fail to address the root cause of the problem, which is a complex and outdated care delivery system. The solution is to restructure the care delivery system because hospitals have become bureaucratic institutions that are no longer able to offer the best possible care to their patients.

Hospital leaders are charged with managing overworked and overburdened healthcare professionals attending to patients in overcrowded hospitals. These healthcare professionals are striving to care for patients who are sicker than ever before and consequently require extremely complex treatments. These treatments in turn require increased documentation for reimbursement of rendered services, all of which prevents these professionals from properly caring for their patients. It is no mystery why healthcare is fraught with waste in this type of environment. It is also easy to recognize the level of desire and dedication necessary to address these issues and eliminate the associated waste.

Changing a hospital's care delivery system requires commitment, vigilance, the ability to make difficult decisions, and unwavering fortitude to withstand intimidation and adversity from those who do not want to change. It also necessitates a different organizational culture. In this book, cultural change does not mean greater camaraderie and affiliation (although these attributes are highly desirable and necessary to any organization's success). Rather, it means development of a culture centered on patients' needs and on providing the best possible care. In such a culture, any circumstance that might jeopardize quality or patient safety is immediately addressed and resolved to eradicate any possibility of reoccurrence; any inefficiency that could delay or otherwise hamper the prompt and appropriate delivery of care to the patient is rectified. It is the culture all healthcare providers aspire to embrace but are repeatedly forced to abandon because of the pressing demands on their time and energy engendered by the structure and focus of the existing care delivery system.

Lean, when properly implemented, creates a customer-focused culture. Contrary to popular belief, Lean is not achieved simply by eliminating wasteful process steps. Derived from the Toyota Production System, Lean is a methodology centered on making every facet of a business work in harmony for the benefit of its customers. Lean organizations produce quality products, recognize their employees as their greatest asset, and constantly pursue perfection in everything they do.

This book is not for hospitals looking for quick fixes or easy solutions or wishing to delegate responsibility. Hospital leaders must confront the inadequacies of the existing care delivery system head-on and oversee the challenging task of creating a Lean enterprise. This endeavor will be arduous and results may not be immediately evident, but perseverance will yield unrivaled success and real healthcare reform.

A Lean Implementation Model

CHAPTER 1

Death by Kaizen Event

We always hope for the easy fix: the one simple change that will erase a problem in a stroke. But few things in life work this way.

—Atul Gawande

Real healthcare reform cannot be legislated. Legislation will not guarantee high-quality care, will not prevent medical errors, and will not promote a more efficient and effective care delivery system. Chronic problems in the healthcare system are plaguing US hospitals, and the finger of blame is pointing in every direction. Hospital administrators, government officials, insurance providers, pharmaceutical companies, and even doctors and nurses have been blamed for the problems associated with healthcare. The blame does not lie with an organization or an individual, however, but with the complex and outdated care delivery system that has been allowed to persist. Every day in every hospital, this system becomes even more complex and more outdated. Therefore, real healthcare reform can come only from within each individual hospital.

There are no silver bullets for chronic problems. It is our nature to want to believe that they exist, but they do not. Still, the peddling of panaceas for almost any problem imaginable has become a lucrative business. We are bombarded every day by television commercials, print advertisements, and billboards soliciting sales of quick fixes for almost all of life's problems. Diet plans promise that you will shed pounds while continuing to eat whatever you desire. Exercise equipment manufacturers promise six-pack abs and hard bodies with minimum effort. Advertisers sell videos promising to have you playing the guitar or speaking a foreign language in just two weeks. Some financial coaches promise to make you wealthy almost overnight. We know that these claims are marketing tactics, yet we allow ourselves to be convinced again and again that the next new product will be different and will deliver the promised results. Almost every home in America has exercise equipment, how-to videos, or self-help books sitting around collecting dust.

All these advertised solutions are designed to solve difficult problems, but they are not quick fixes; they are presented in a way that makes you think that they are. Many of these marketing claims are true, but only if the plan or product is applied correctly and given sufficient time to produce the desired results. You will lose weight while eating what you want if you eat smaller portions and do not snack between meals. Exercise equipment will tone your body, but only if you do the exercises correctly and consistently and eat a proper diet. You might even become a millionaire overnight if the conditions are just right and you follow the prescribed steps meticulously. The resolution of chronic problems requires discipline, tenacity, precise execution, and hard work.

Healthcare is experiencing difficult times as a result of chronic problems. Reimbursements are declining, the costs of supplies and pharmaceuticals are rising, inpatient facilities are losing revenue to outpatient centers, healthcare workers are commanding high salaries as a result of the healthcare labor shortage, and the cost of malpractice insurance is steep. In addition, there are quality issues resulting from adverse medical events, inefficiencies, system breakdowns, medication errors, and ineffective standards. Hospital leaders are overwhelmed, staff are overworked, and doctors are overburdened; they all want and need relief, and they want it quickly.

Lean can provide this relief, but contrary to what many organizational leaders have been led to believe, Lean is not a quick fix, is not easy, cannot be delegated, cannot be purchased, cannot be done piecemeal, and cannot be consultant driven. To generate the desired outcome, Lean must be implemented correctly and consistently and be given sufficient time. Everyone in the organization must commit to becoming Lean. It requires strategically directed action, creation of a Lean organizational culture, and redesign of the organization's care delivery system. In short, Lean is serious business.

The obvious question at this juncture is: Why would an overwhelmed, overworked, and overburdened hospital want to engage a methodology that requires even more from them? The answer is simple: There are no quick fixes for the problems hospitals face, and purposeful effort is the only way to make things better. If hospitals do not take the action necessary to improve healthcare, it will most assuredly get worse, and hospital leadership cannot afford to let that happen.

We are a results-driven society. We want results, and we want them now. Quick results are the pervasive goal in our multitasking, hyperactive existence. Computers deliver information in nanoseconds, we eat fast food, and we take fast-acting pain relievers. Our careers are on the fast track, we drive fast cars in the fast lane, and we make split-second decisions. We look for shortcuts and tend to skip vital steps in an effort to experience benefits sooner.

This inherent desire for quick results drives organizational leaders to attempt to "purchase" Lean and forgo the critical steps necessary for successful Lean implementation. Leaders dive in headfirst and immediately experience the benefits associated with Lean by conducting as many *kaizen* events (i.e., kaizen blitz or rapid improvement events) as they can in the shortest time frame, with little regard for the prerequisites. These expensive campaigns of kaizen events inevitably culminate by imposing changes on staff members. The improvements prompted by each event are impressive, but they are often short lived. Many Lean concepts are counterintuitive, and unless staff understand and internalize Lean principles, they will abandon these imposed improvements and revert to their old work habits. Consequently, performance returns to its previous level. If Lean could be purchased and quickly and easily achieved, every organization would be Lean, just as we would all be wealthy, talented people with rock-hard bodies. Lean is not a silver bullet, an easy fix, or a magic potion. Creating a Lean organization entails hard work, but if Lean is implemented correctly, the return on investment will exceed leaders' expectations.

By skipping the critical steps necessary for success, organizations fail to lay a solid foundation on which to build a Lean enterprise. Instead, they create an illusion of success. Consider the classic Lean implementation practice of conducting a series of kaizen events. First, the senior administrators select the events. The following categories are the most common selection criteria:

- The greatest problem area
- Low-hanging fruit (problems that can be solved with minimum effort)
- Areas in which the staff would be most open to change
- The area that will yield the most return on investment

Unknowingly, the organization is already off to a poor start. Such initiatives have no strategic basis, nor do they build on previous successes. Instead, they target superficial issues that are the symptoms of a much bigger problem. In medicine, addressing symptoms and ignoring the cause of those symptoms could result in irreparable damage or death. Likewise, with Lean, addressing symptoms rather than causes could result in irreparable damage to the organization or death of the Lean initiative.

When manufacturing companies began implementing Lean, the accepted method was to conduct a series of kaizen events to address problem areas. Pre-event training typically comprised a one- to two-hour session in which participants built airplanes out of Lego blocks and spent the majority of the remaining time learning to use Lean worksheets. This training provided only a rudimentary introduction to Lean and did little to advance participants' understanding of Lean principles.

Next the organization would engage a consultant or in-house facilitator to facilitate the kaizen events. Upon completion of the event, managers, supervisors, and workers were left to sustain the improvements and close out any open items on their own. Without the facilitator's guidance and lacking an in-depth understanding of Lean principles, these individuals struggled to maintain the proposed improvements and in many cases resisted the changes. They became bogged down in their attempts to apply Lean tools, and departments' disagreements over assignment of responsibilities provoked turf wars. Staff became discouraged, more urgent matters took priority, and departments slowly reverted to the methods they understood and were comfortable using. Eventually, department performance returned to its previous level.

Consequently, the kaizen event became a new category of waste in the minds of staff members. They considered the time, effort, and resources dedicated to a weeklong initiative an even greater waste than the waste associated with the targeted problem. Adding to this lack of acceptance was senior level management's determination to implement more and more kaizen events. This persistence induced only higher levels of resistance, lower morale, and a negative attitude toward the Lean methodology.

Ultimately, Lean became something to avoid rather than embrace. As a result of the kaizen blitz implementation strategy, many more manufacturing organizations failed than succeeded in their Lean efforts. In November 2007, *Industry Week* released the results of its Industry Week/Manufacturing Performance Institute (IW/MPI) Census of Manufacturers. The IW/MPI report showed that 70 percent of the manufacturing companies surveyed were currently employing Lean manufacturing as an improvement methodology but that less than a quarter (24 percent) of those companies reported achieving significant results from their Lean implementation; a mere 2 percent indicated that they achieved their objective of becoming a Lean organization. The remaining 74 percent were achieving less than significant results not because Lean is not an effective improvement methodology but because they were not implementing it properly.

THE NUMMI EXPERIMENT

In 1984 General Motors entered into a joint venture with Toyota. Together they reopened one of General Motors' manufacturing plants in Fremont, California. The joint venture was called New United Motor Manufacturing Incorporated, better known as NUMMI. General Motors' motivation to enter the venture was to learn about Lean manufacturing from Toyota. Toyota's incentive was to test whether its manufacturing methods would be accepted in a Western culture.

The United Auto Workers Union had identified the workers at the former Fremont plant as the "worst workforce in the automobile industry in the United States" (National Public Radio 2010). Excessive absenteeism, drinking on the job, sexual relations at the plant, and petty acts of sabotage were common occurrences. Shutdown of the production line was considered taboo, and defects were permitted to continue along the assembly line, to be fixed later. Many of these same workers were rehired when the NUMMI plant reopened in 1984.

Toyota executives did not implement Lean by conducting a series of kaizen events and force-feeding the methodology to this workforce. Instead they educated the workers in Lean principles to promote a thorough understanding of the concepts. These workers then put Lean to work on the production floor. Almost immediately, the quality of both Toyota and General Motors automobiles built at the NUMMI plant rivaled the quality of those built at Toyota plants in Japan. Following its successes at NUMMI,

Toyota went on to build Toyota Motor Manufacturing Kentucky (TMMK) in Georgetown, Kentucky, Toyota's first wholly owned manufacturing facility in the United States. TMMK produces approximately 500,000 quality vehicles every year.

General Motors, however, attempted to implement Lean tools at its other factories in the United States without first training the workforce in Lean principles and failed to generate the results achieved at the NUMMI plant. In 2009 General Motors requested and received a $50 billion government bailout to emerge from bankruptcy. Learning about Lean tools from Toyota, the developers of the Toyota Production System, was not enough to ensure General Motors' success. Use of Lean tools alone, no matter how well management understands them or how often they are implemented, does not guarantee success. Success with Lean requires cultural change and a system focus.

Healthcare cannot afford to make the same mistakes that General Motors and so many other manufacturing companies have made. There are no quick fixes, and organizations will not achieve results faster by skipping steps. To be successful, hospital leaders must roll up their sleeves and do what is necessary to create a true Lean enterprise.

THE FIRST REALIZATION REGARDING LEAN

Too many organizations view Lean as a set of tools used to improve processes by eliminating wasteful process steps and creating flow, but Lean is much more than a set of tools. The tools merely facilitate the implementation; they are a means to an end and are secondary to Lean principles. If the organization applying the tools does not understand and practice Lean principles, the successes resulting from kaizen events will be superficial and short lived.

Everyone in the organization needs to understand basic Lean concepts; this knowledge is not reserved for senior or middle management. The ultimate goal is to establish a Lean culture—a culture in which all staff members are constantly on the lookout for opportunities to identify and correct inconsistencies in their processes, establish systems that enable timely and accurate execution of their duties, and recognize and eliminate constraints to the delivery of patient care.

In organizations that do not have a Lean culture, improvements proposed in kaizen events will fail to take hold. In a Lean culture, improvements occur daily or even hourly. Although they may seem minor and insubstantial, these improvements are significant and, even more important, sustainable, and staff experience the benefits of Lean firsthand.

THE SECOND REALIZATION REGARDING LEAN

Lean is not a firefighting methodology. Kaizen events are often scheduled to address problem areas. However, kaizen events should be identified and scheduled with the goal of creating flow through the entire process, which in Lean terminology is referred to as the *value stream*. The value stream often crosses departmental boundaries and may comprise six or more departments. Organizations commonly need to conduct several kaizen events to establish flow through the entire process defined by the desired (future) state of the value stream.

Unless the value stream's support functions, such as diagnostic imaging, laboratory services, and transport, are involved in kaizen events, the benefits will be unsustainable. Support functions are commonly identified as constraints to flow, and changes are made, or steps are added, to their processes with little or no input from them. By revising their processes, the kaizen team is "throwing waste over the wall"—i.e., shifting responsibility for wasteful process steps from one department to another. This transfer of responsibility clearly does not constitute an improvement. Constraints to flow must be resolved, not merely reassigned. For example, if the emergency department (ED) feels that it wastes too much time transporting patients to the diagnostic imaging (DI) department, it might assign the transport responsibility to DI staff. DI then has to add transport to its staff members' responsibilities. By shifting the transport responsibility from the ED to DI, the ED has thrown waste over the wall. Therefore, support functions must understand and take an active role in working toward the desired state of the value stream.

Lean is a system, and as such it requires systems thinking. The organization must identify the value stream, including all support functions; define the outcome it is seeking to achieve; create a plan detailing how it will achieve that desired state; assign accountability for plan outcomes to all departments; and finally, execute the plan. When Lean is approached in this manner, each kaizen event builds on the successes of the previous event, thereby creating flow through the entire process.

THE KEY TO SUCCESS

Lean has the potential to transform healthcare, but like most things worth having, it comes with a price. This price has both a monetary and a nonmonetary component. The monetary component is the actual dollars spent to implement the Lean methodology. Because Lean focuses on simple and inexpensive improvement methods as opposed to innovative change, this cost is minimal. The nonmonetary component is the time and resources devoted to Lean implementation and the risk that the methodology will not deliver the expected benefits.

The objective, therefore, is to minimize this risk and maximize the likelihood of success through proper implementation, commitment, action, and support. Do not skip steps; identify and take immediate action to resolve problems and eliminate waste; and support the provision of necessary resources. As the expected benefits are realized, the monetary and nonmonetary costs of Lean implementation will diminish. Hospitals will generate less waste, have fewer problems, and commit fewer errors. Employee morale will improve, costs will decrease, and revenue will increase. Staff will be able to devote more time and resources to other value-adding activities, such as technological advancement. Most important, hospitals will deliver better patient care.

It is recommended that an organization retain a consultant for guidance through the implementation process. However, be leery of consulting firms that expound on the savings and process improvements they have generated for their clients. In an organization that has failed to first create a Lean culture and internalize the concept of systems thinking, the gains such firms describe are seldom realized; rather, they are describing the savings the organization might have experienced had it sustained the consultant's imposed changes. Furthermore, for consulting firms to take credit for these savings and improvements is inappropriate. The consultant's job is to educate the staff and guide the organization through the implementation process, not to impose change. Imposed change will not transform a hospital into a Lean enterprise; the change must come from within the organization. Bottom-up implementation is essential to sustained improvement.

In summary, there are two components to successful Lean implementation. The first is creation of a Lean culture. The second is elimination of departmental boundaries and flow through the care delivery system. Everyone in the organization must understand that the hospital is a system, and that for a system to function properly, all of its parts must work together.

Many organizations struggle with the dilemma of which to create first: a Lean culture or a system. They are struggling needlessly; the culture and the system are intertwined and are implemented together. The following chapters will guide you through a model for successful Lean implementation.

SUMMARY: Death by Kaizen Event

- Lean is not a quick fix, is not easy, cannot be delegated, cannot be purchased, cannot be done piecemeal, and cannot be consultant driven.

- By skipping the critical steps necessary for success, organizations fail to lay a solid foundation on which to build their Lean enterprise.

- The ultimate goal is to establish a Lean culture, in which all staff members are constantly on the lookout for opportunities to identify and correct inconsistencies in their processes, establish systems that enable timely and accurate execution of their duties, and recognize and eliminate constraints to the delivery of patient care.

- Lean is a system, and as such it requires systems thinking. Organizations must identify the value stream, including all support functions; define the outcome they are seeking to achieve; create a plan detailing how they will achieve that desired state; assign accountability for plan outcomes to all departments; and finally, execute the plan.

CHAPTER 2

A Lean Implementation Model

There is nothing more uncommon than common sense.
—Frank Lloyd Wright

When presented in the appropriate context, many Lean concepts are simply common sense—shared practical judgment. However, we often do not use common sense because it is the path of greatest resistance. Common sense dictates that waste is undesirable and should be eliminated at every opportunity, but we accept waste as circumstantial. Common sense tells us that mistakes should be reported and immediate action should be taken to identify and eliminate their root causes, yet we address mistakes superficially and in many cases do not even report them. It is common sense to remove departmental boundaries and other obstacles that impede flow, but instead we add steps to an already complex process to work around these obstructions rather than deal with them directly.

Waiting rooms are constructed to accommodate patients at value stream bottlenecks. Nurses are responsible for stocking, counting, and maintaining proper supply levels. Overcrowded emergency departments are treating patients in hallways devoid of privacy. These processes have been put in place because they appeared to be the best way to handle the immediate problem. At the time, they seemed reasonable, logical, and expedient. In reality, they were reactive, results-driven, quick fixes imposed with little thought or communication and implemented with the goal of attracting as little attention as possible by minimizing disruption to daily operations. The focus was not on solving the problem but on dealing with the situation and getting everyone back to work as quickly as possible.

Instead of promoting productivity, however, quick fixes impede it. They often add work for the staff and leave the door wide open for errors to occur. The need to handle the situation as expeditiously as possible overrides any impulse we have to take a commonsensical approach and spend the time necessary to properly address the root cause of the problem. It is easy to see how these quick fixes, defined in Lean terms as *layers*, create more complexity and increase the likelihood of errors.

Because Lean concepts do not prescribe easy fixes, staff easily revert to using the methods they have used during most of their working lives. The following story from my own experience demonstrates this tendency. Working as a manufacturing manager, I was responsible for the assembly of several products manufactured by my employer. Two hardworking, conscientious women assembled one of these products. Using the "batch and queue" method for assembling this product, they would jointly produce 25 assemblies per day. Despite all my efforts to convince them that "one-piece flow" would generate more parts and result in fewer defects, they continued to batch. One morning, I decided to try a little experiment. I let them assemble the products using batching for half a day. At lunchtime there were 25 assemblies halfway through the process. After lunch I asked them to put the 25 semi-completed assemblies to the side and work the rest of the day making one product at a time from the beginning of the process. At the end of the day, they had jointly completed 22 assemblies, all defect-free—almost a full day's production completed in half a day. Finally, they were convinced that one-piece flow was better than batch and queue. Every time I walked by their assembly line, they were busily assembling products one at a time. Production went up, and defects went down. I thought I had converted the women until one day, while walking by their line, I noticed they were batching again. When I inquired as to why they abandoned one-piece flow, they told me they were working on a rush job and had to get it done quickly.

These women never really appreciated the true value of one-piece flow. When the pressure was on to expedite production, they reverted to their comfortable and familiar method of batch and queue. This backslide is a normal response to stressful situations. Backsliding is common and is a major frustration for individuals responsible for implementing process improvement initiatives. Sometimes the methods and improvements put in place to establish flow appear to impede efficiency at a departmental level, but they are often necessary to create flow through the value stream. It is counterproductive to abandon Lean concepts and revert to previously established methods because they are easier or more comfortable to use. An organization cannot become a true Lean enterprise unless staff understand the value of Lean tools and concepts.

People need time to acclimate to change, even simple change. Dr. Maxwell Maltz, author of the bestselling book *Psycho-Cybernetics: A New Way to Get More Living Out of Life* (1960), demonstrated that it takes almost exactly three weeks to develop a habit. This time frame is a useful gauge when implementing change. If after 21 days the change still does not feel right, do not impulsively declare the improvement effort a failure. Reevaluate the situation; look for anomalies, such as disproportionate par levels for supplies, unbalanced process steps, or unforeseen delays; and take appropriate action to eliminate them. The efficacy of Lean tools and concepts has been proven many times over; allow time for change to take effect.

THE IMPLEMENTATION MODEL

Common sense advocates a quality focus to establish organizational stability, yet financially motivated mandates and projects are routinely introduced instead. Many people believe that it costs more to provide quality service than to provide average or substandard service. This belief is a fallacy. Superior quality costs much less than poor quality. Higher quality means better care for the patient and lower costs for the organization. Revenue less costs equals net income, so lower costs mean higher net income. Higher net income enables an organization to provide more and better services, thereby creating new jobs and a greater level of job security for its employees. Excellence through quality is a win-win-win venture: The patient receives the best possible care, the organization prospers, and everyone in the organization has reason to feel a sense of worth and security.

A Lean transformation does not occur in some organizations and fail in others because of sheer luck or desire alone. The key to a successful Lean transformation is proper implementation. An overly aggressive and demanding management team that imposes change on staff members by conducting consultant-driven kaizen events and haphazardly implementing Lean tools will create only an illusion of success.

Proper implementation means the organization must adhere to an established implementation model. This model must provide strategic direction relative to improvements to the care delivery system and establish a Lean culture at the same time. In addition, the implementation model must be somewhat flexible to accommodate unforeseen obstacles or setbacks but at the same time be structurally sound and chart an unambiguous path to success.

The model illustrated in Exhibit 2.1 incorporates these characteristics and simultaneously implements two distinct paths that lead to the common objective of creating a Lean enterprise. The two paths originate with the organization's strategic plan and cascade toward organizational transformation via a quality culture and an enhanced care delivery system. The path to the right in Exhibit 2.1 is the culture-creating path, which engenders a learning/action-taking organization in which disclosure of problems, continuous improvement, and empowerment become standard operating procedure. The path to the left in Exhibit 2.1 is the system-creating path, which provides strategic direction for Lean implementation and focuses on creating flow through the strategically identified value streams by eliminating barriers, reducing inventory, and leveling the process.

These two paths are interdependent, meaning that the benefits experienced in one path are dependent on the proper execution of the other path. Both are equally critical to creating a Lean enterprise; an attempt to execute one while disregarding the other will not produce the desired outcome. This point cannot be overemphasized.

Exhibit 2.1: Zidel's Model for Lean Implementation

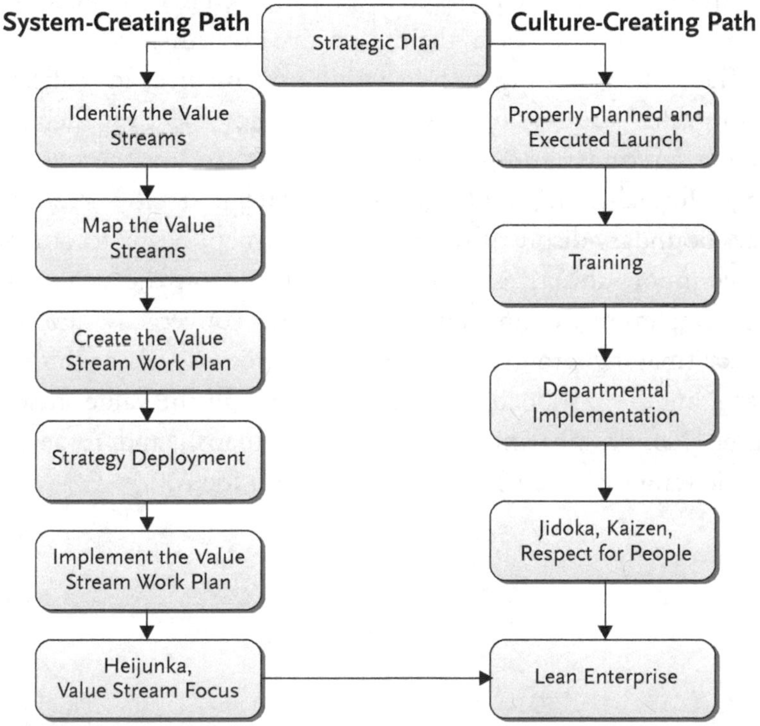

Regrettably, most Lean initiatives focus on one of the two paths and neglect the other, or they give disingenuous attention to one while concentrating all efforts on the other. Too often neither path is followed. In these cases, kaizen events and short-term wins are the focal points of implementation.

The culture-creating path illustrated in Exhibit 2.1 promotes Lean transformation by teaching staff to solve problems. Training is the most important step to changing an organizational culture, as demonstrated by the NUMMI joint venture described in Chapter 1. Too often new programs are launched without proper instruction. Lack of training leads to confusion about proper application of Lean tools, misinterpretation of Lean concepts, indifference about the success of the Lean transformation, and, eventually, failure of the initiative. Before change can take hold, people must understand the proposed culture and know what will be expected of them. Upon completion of training, management and staff are instructed to experiment with Lean tools and concepts in their respective departments.

The system-creating path in Exhibit 2.1 involves identification of the value streams implicated in strategic objectives, depicting the current and future state of these value streams, and creating a plan for achieving the future state. Strategic deployment eliminates boundary disputes by making department heads accountable for common objectives. Kaizen events build on the successes of preceding events. Ultimately, the two paths converge, synthesizing jidoka (making problems obvious), heijunka (level loading [i.e., managing the workload to create flow through the value stream]), kaizen (continuous incremental improvement), and respect for people (empowerment) with a value stream focus.

SUMMARY: A Lean Implementation Model

- Lean tools and principles are common sense.

- For a Lean transformation to be successful, the organization must develop and adhere to an implementation strategy. This strategy implements two paths simultaneously:
    - The culture-creating path engenders a learning/action-taking organization in which making problems obvious, continuous improvement, and empowerment become standard operating procedure.
    - The system-creating path provides strategic direction for Lean implementation and focuses on creating flow through the strategically identified value streams by eliminating barriers, reducing inventory levels, and leveling flow.

CHAPTER 3

Strategically Directed Action

Vision without action is a dream. Action without vision is simply pass-ing the time. Action with vision is making a positive difference.
—Joel Baker

The Lean implementation model illustrated in Exhibit 2.1 begins with a strategic plan. Strategically directed action is essential to achieving an organization's goals. A strategic plan is a forward-looking plan that clearly defines what an organization does and identifies objectives it must achieve to perform better. Hospitals' objectives usually entail providing better quality care, more effi-ciently, without errors, and cost effectively. Naturally, the specif-ics of how an organization plans to accomplish its objectives are dependent on many factors unique to it. Size, location, competi-tion, and community are just a few of those factors.

Almost all hospitals have a strategic plan. At some point, a hospital's senior leadership team likely spent a week or more off-site deliberating the organization's strategic focus. The team analyzed the hospital's strengths, weaknesses, opportunities, and threats prior to developing the plan. It probably spent hours formulating a plan that would capitalize on those strengths, minimize perceived threats, take advantage of identified oppor-tunities, and integrate defensive tactics to deemphasize apparent weaknesses. At some point prior to the strategy planning session, this group presumably labored for days, weeks, or perhaps months developing mission, vision, and values statements for the hospital. Respectively, the mission, vision, and values statements answer the questions "What do we do?", "What do we want to become?", and "What are our priorities?"

All this time and hard work were not in vain. On the contrary, the effort was an extremely important undertaking and time well spent. All organizations must understand their core competencies, identify their priorities, and have detailed long- and short-term plans to help them meet their strategic objectives. Without strategic direction, a hospital will continuously struggle in its attempts to improve or even to remain a viable asset to its patients. Misdirected organizations (or those lacking a strategic focus) jump around, launch one initiative after another, and succeed only in confusing their staffs and increasing resistance to change. These organizations epitomize the old saying "If you don't know where you're going, any road will take you there."

If a hospital does not have a current strategic plan, its leaders need to develop one. Most organizations already have a strategic plan and just need to update it. Plan development/revision usually necessitates some time off-site, away from the daily tasks and interruptions of a normal workday. Leaders are advised to solicit the assistance of a strategic planning expert to guide them through this process.

COMMITMENT

As is true with any organizational change initiative, the most essential ingredient for a successful Lean transformation is the commitment of the senior leadership team. A lack of commitment allowed to persist unchallenged on the part of any member of the senior leadership team will undoubtedly cause the transformation to fail. A senior leader's lack of enthusiasm regarding the Lean initiative will indicate to his direct reports that he considers Lean just another of the many methodologies adopted by the hospital, and like the others, it will soon be abandoned only to have a new program quickly take its place.

If the administrative team does not actively demonstrate support for Lean, staff will not take the initiative seriously and counteracting forces will sabotage attempts to improve. Managers will revert to a departmental focus (as opposed to a strategic focus) and prioritize their personal (or departmental) agendas over the organization's needs. As a result, bureaucracy will bog down quality initiatives, and any improvements resulting from quality projects will be allowed to regress, thereby negating efforts. Eventually, staff will recognize the futility of their efforts to improve, and slowly but surely, they will stop trying.

The importance of the entire leadership team's enthusiastic support of the initiative cannot be overemphasized. Ultimately, every member of the organization must develop an equivalent commitment to quality. This commitment is best learned through example, and for this reason the organization's message must be reinforced with actions. For senior leaders, active participation in the Lean transformation may include conducting morning rounds, developing rapport with staff members, becoming a visible presence in the organization, providing necessary resources for Lean projects, attending final presentation of kaizen events, giving regular feedback to staff, and doggedly pursuing excellence through quality. Any actions that are contrary to or inconsistent with their verbal message are detrimental and could undermine the development of a Lean culture. This responsibility is enormous, but organizational leadership is an enormous responsibility.

The chief executive officer or any other member of the senior leadership team alone, no matter how competent, rarely possesses all the assets necessary to overcome every obstacle encountered in a Lean transformation. The effort must be amalgamated to be successful. Furthermore, the senior leadership team must be a cohesive group. Dissension, lack of trust, or disrespect among team members will guarantee failure. This team must be united in its dedication to providing high-quality patient care and exhibit a mutual desire to do what is best for the organization.

STRATEGIC VERSUS TACTICAL IMPLEMENTATION

Many organizational leaders get excited about Lean. They want to implement Lean tools and reap benefits as soon as possible. More than likely they have a handful of issues that have been in queue awaiting rectification for some time, and they can't wait to unleash the powers of Lean and watch their problems magically disappear. With inflated expectations they schedule their first kaizen event and wait with optimistic eagerness for the final presentation so they can see firsthand the outcome of the Lean team's weeklong assignment.

The final presentation progresses as the team announces its objectives, explains the situation before the event, describes its accomplishments, and presents the situation after the event. Finally, it enumerates the benefits the organization has reaped from the event. Increased revenue, decreased costs, enhanced patient satisfaction, quicker turnaround times, and other positive indicators are proudly displayed for everyone present. The team likely has met or exceeded all expectations. All in attendance at the final presentation are appropriately impressed. They applaud the team's efforts, and representatives from senior leadership communicate the hospital's sincere appreciation for a job well done.

This demonstration is a typical and appropriate end to a kaizen event. However, tactically scheduled kaizen events such as that just described are by far the most consequential aberration from proper implementation of Lean. Organization leaders are not intimately involved in the process, so they are lulled into complacency regarding the initiative. They continue to schedule events with the same tactical motivation, unable or unwilling to recognize that these events are not moving them any closer to their strategic objectives.

Each event demands precious time and resources from staff members who seldom experience the promised benefits.

An organization that schedules kaizen events around problems will not become a Lean enterprise. The number and frequency of such events also have no bearing on whether it achieves transformation. Implementations targeted at solving problems are rarely linked to the strategic plan and are conducted to mitigate highly visible issues in the organization, such as overcrowding of the emergency department, medication errors, or slow turnarounds on lab tests. In short, the organization reduces Lean to a firefighting tool. In some cases, the outcomes of these events may be notable; the organization's leaders are impressed, articles are written and published, presentations are conducted at conferences, and best practices may be established. However, the organization has minimized only a segment of a much bigger problem, and the bigger problem will certainly persist.

Strategically directed implementation is the critical first step to enhancing the overall service delivery process of the identified value stream. Knowledge of the hospital's strategic objectives and effort directed toward those goals are fundamental to a true Lean enterprise. Exhibit 3.1 contrasts tactical and strategic motivation.

Exhibit 3.1: Tactical Versus Strategic Motivation for Kaizen Events

Tactical	Strategic
Short-term focus (present)	Long-term focus (future)
Reactive (firefighting)	Proactive (fire prevention)
Small change	Big change
How to fix it	Why it is broken
Focus on a problem	Focus on an opportunity
Lacks linkage to other events	Builds on previous successes
Quick fix	Sustainable quality improvement

Strategically directed action is the difference between Lean implementation and Lean transformation. Lean tools implemented without the direction supplied by a strategic focus are themselves a source of waste: wasted effort, wasted money, and wasted time.

SUMMARY: Strategically Directed Action

- The most essential ingredient for a successful Lean transformation is the commitment of the senior leadership team.

- Tactically scheduled kaizen events are the most consequential aberration from proper implementation of Lean.

- Strategically directed implementation is the critical first step to enhancing the overall service delivery process of the identified value stream.

- Strategically directed action is the difference between Lean implementation and Lean transformation.

CREATING A LEAN CULTURE

CHAPTER 4

The Culture-Creating Path

Quality is the result of a carefully constructed cultural environment.
—Phillip Crosby

Culture is the environment derived from a set of implied understandings shared by the people who work in an organization. It determines how people interact with one another and with individuals outside the organization. Culture is formed from past experiences, basic assumptions, beliefs, attitudes, and existing behaviors. Culture change is extremely difficult and requires time, patience, and commitment. The culture-creating path of the Lean implementation model illustrated in Exhibit 4.1 identifies the elements necessary to effect organizational culture change. Essentially, the purposes of the three steps—launch, training, and implementation—are to inform, educate, and apply.

LAUNCH

The launch of the Lean initiative should be properly planned and executed to inform staff of the answers to these questions:

- What is Lean?
- Where is it being implemented?

Exhibit 4.1: The Culture-Creating Path of the Lean Implementation Model

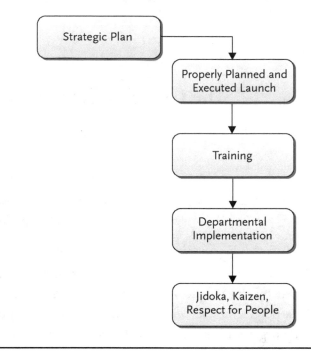

- Why is the organization adopting this methodology?
- When will implementation begin?
- How will it proceed?

A properly planned and executed launch also demonstrates the commitment of senior administration to the Lean initiative.

TRAINING

Training is provided to educate all, not just key, staff members in Lean principles and tools. Many times hospital leaders identify individuals and send them to workshops to learn Lean. This approach is fine if the goal is to help the organization decide whether to adopt Lean as an improvement methodology. However, if the goal is to have these individuals return from the workshop and begin implementing what they have learned, the leaders are making a big mistake. By implementing what they have learned, these individuals are essentially imposing change, and imposed change will be short lived, regardless of whether a consultant or someone in the organization initiates it. The goal is to teach all staff members to solve problems or know what action to take if they witness something that could jeopardize quality or patient safety. Naturally this training should be commensurate with each individual's level of responsibility in the organization.

IMPLEMENTATION

By implementing Lean at the department level, staff members can apply Lean tools and principles in a familiar and secure environment. Lean is best learned through application, so staff must apply these tools and principles themselves. In a familiar environment, they will be less fearful of making mistakes and experimenting with different concepts. The goal is for staff members to develop a level of comfort with Lean, gain experience with the tools and principles, and witness the benefits of Lean firsthand.

THE HOUSE OF LEAN

A primary focus for any organization embarking on a Lean initiative must be the development of a Lean culture. This culture is the foundation on which the Lean organization will be built. It nurtures quality, provides value to the organization's customers, and teaches employees to solve problems. This culture takes hold when members of the organization internalize the three key elements of Lean: standard work (i.e., standard operating procedure), user-friendliness, and unobstructed throughput.

Building a Lean enterprise is analogous to building a house. For this reason, the elements associated with Lean can be illustrated as a house, commonly referred to as the "House of Lean." There are many variations to the House of Lean, some elaborate and complex. The House of Lean depicted in Exhibit 4.2 is straightforward yet includes all the necessary components for a Lean enterprise. Note that the three elements of standard work, user-friendliness, and unobstructed throughput form the foundation of the house.

Construction of a house must follow a logical sequence to ensure timely completion, minimize problems, and produce the best possible results. The most logical (and only plausible) sequence in which to build a house is to build it from the bottom up. Who would consider constructing a house by starting in the middle or beginning with the roof and working down to the foundation?

This logic is not always as apparent when implementing improvement methodologies in hospitals and other organizations, however. As discussed in Chapter 1, due to an overpowering

Exhibit 4.2: The House of Lean

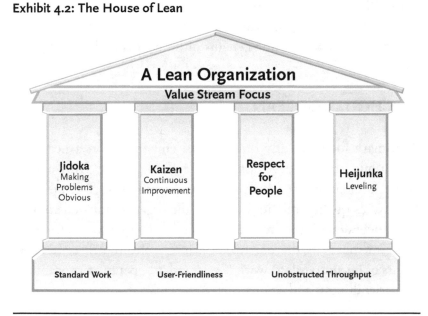

eagerness to witness the implementation of Lean tools and reap the associated benefits, many organizational leaders launch their Lean initiatives by jumping in and conducting kaizen events. This approach is analogous to commencing the construction of a house in the middle. A house without a solid foundation will crumble under the slightest of adverse conditions. The same is true of a Lean initiative. Kaizen events conducted as a platform from which to launch a Lean initiative do much more harm than good. The true benefits of Lean can be realized only by first constructing a solid foundation of Lean culture.

Like the three elements used to construct a strong foundation for a house—cement, sand, and water—the three elements of standard work, user-friendliness, and unobstructed throughput must be competently integrated and exist in concert to solidify a firm foundation for a Lean organization. For example, adherence to standard work is not possible unless the process is user-friendly and throughput is unobstructed. Just as sand or water alone cannot form a foundation, an organization cannot build a Lean foundation from just one or two of these elements.

The care and coordinated effort that go into constructing a Lean organization determine its durability, just as they determine the durability of a house. Without a solid cultural foundation, a Lean initiative is susceptible to outside forces and destined to collapse.

SUMMARY: The Culture-Creating Path

- A primary focus for any organization embarking on a Lean initiative must be the development of a Lean culture.

- This culture necessitates that all members of the organization internalize the three key elements of Lean: standard work, user-friendliness, and unobstructed throughput.

- Without a solid cultural foundation, a Lean initiative is susceptible to outside forces and destined to collapse.

CHAPTER 5

A Properly Planned Launch

Before anything else, preparation is the key to success.
—Alexander Graham Bell

Companies invest a great deal of time and effort planning the launch of new products. The purpose of a launch is to stimulate an awareness of a new product and instill in the target market a desire and readiness to purchase it. Companies create this anticipation by highlighting the product's new features and demonstrating its superiority to earlier or competitors' versions. Often they launch the product months before it becomes available to the public.

Apple Inc. is a perfect example of a company that skillfully develops and executes product launches. It launches its new products, often six months or more prior to release, at highly publicized media events at its Cupertino, California, campus. At these conferences the company reveals new features that up until the launch it had alluded to but not confirmed. It stimulates so much excitement and anticipation for its new products that some customers sleep outside Apple stores the night prior to the products' release so they do not miss the opportunity to purchase them. Not surprisingly, the stores often sell out of the new product early in the day.

An organization is unlikely to be able to generate this same level of enthusiasm for an improvement program, but failure to properly launch a Lean initiative can, and most likely will, have the opposite effect. Instead of anticipation, desire, and readiness, the new program will generate apprehension, indifference, and avoidance.

Without a formal introduction to the Lean initiative, staff will derive most of what they know about Lean from rumors or sources outside the organization. What they hear might be positive, but it could be negative, and it is human nature to believe the bad and question the good. If staff do not receive information or answers to their questions about the new initiative, they will make assumptions. They will assume that Lean will benefit the organization but not necessarily be good for them or their patients. They will assume that the new program will require additional work and leave them with less time to perform their regular duties. They will assume that they will be the only ones required to change while everyone else reaps the benefits of their efforts. And they will assume that the term *Lean* means people will be laid off. Rumors will circulate through the organization, bolstering these assumptions and escalating the staff's level of apprehension. As a result, the staff will take on a defensive attitude and oppose any efforts to change. They will conjure up reasons why Lean won't work in their department or concoct scenarios in which Lean implementation will generate complications or negative ramifications. Senior leadership will then have to force change on the organization to drive individuals from their comfort zones. This type of introduction to Lean is seldom, if ever, successful. Regrettably, many organizations begin their Lean transformation with an uninformed, anxious, and cynical staff.

Senior leaders seldom give serious consideration, if any, to the launch of a new quality program. Most often programs are initiated without any formal announcement, or at best they begin via an e-mail blast from the CEO. The message usually includes rudimentary information about the program and ends with a statement such as "I know I can count on all of you to support this initiative, and I'm looking forward to seeing some great things." Such announcements do little to create excitement about the new program. Rather, they usually create anxiety in an already overburdened staff, who interpret the announcement as a notification of yet another item to add to their long lists of things to do rather than as an opportunity to make things better.

A properly planned and implemented launch prepares the staff for what is to follow, thereby minimizing cultural resistance, surprises, and the circulation of assumptions and rumors. A mass mailing from the CEO to all members of the organization is an acceptable start, but it must be followed by a more formal launch that will offer everyone in the organization an opportunity to learn and ask questions. For example, an organization could reserve one of its regularly scheduled "state of the hospital" meetings for the formal launch.

It is advisable to begin the launch with some background information that segues to the topic of Lean. Many experts in the field of change recommend creating a sense of urgency, but this step is not necessary in healthcare because a sense of urgency already pervades the industry. Similarly, presentation of reams of financial data to demonstrate that the hospital is operating at a loss can render the audience apathetic from the beginning. Open the launch with an incentive that staff can relate to and that is near and dear to them: their patients. Patients are the reason most people chose to work in healthcare. The desire to provide high-quality care is intrinsic to hospital staff members. When they are prevented from providing what they consider an appropriate level of patient care, they become frustrated, annoyed, or angry, so the prospect of eliminating barriers to providing high-quality patient care is an ideal platform from which to launch a Lean transformation. This incentive is a venture that staff members can rally around. Such an opening will capture everyone's attention and make the audience anxious to learn more.

It is important to make crystal clear from the beginning that Lean targets wasteful processes and not people. Now over a decade old, the Institute of Medicine (IOM) report, *To Err Is Human: Building a Safer Health System* (2000) estimated that "98,000 people die annually from medical errors which could have been prevented." This sentence suggests that healthcare workers are incompetent, irresponsible, and perhaps even malicious. The IOM report did not intend to make this suggestion. The intent was to raise awareness about the need to change the care delivery system. The report goes on to declare that

> The majority of medical errors do not result from individual recklessness or the actions of a particular group—this is not a "bad apple" problem. More commonly, errors are caused by faulty systems, processes, and conditions that lead people to make mistakes or fail to prevent them.

These faulty systems, processes, and conditions are the target of Lean.

Another key element at the launch and at subsequent progress meetings is the presence of all members of the senior leadership team. Their attendance will demonstrate their united support of the Lean initiative. The absence of these individuals communicates to the staff that the initiative is something the staff must engage in, but not senior management. If the staff and middle management witness a lack of commitment on the part of senior management, they may deem the initiative "the flavor of the month" before it even gets off the ground.

THE ORGANIZATIONAL HIERARCHY FOR LEAN IMPLEMENTATION

Staff members' roles in the Lean initiative should also be clarified at the launch. Top-down commitment is essential to the successful creation of a Lean organization, but equally important is the concept of bottom-up implementation. It is essential that Lean implementation involve the participation of frontline staff and that change is not imposed from the top down.

The organizational hierarchy for Lean implementation turns the traditional hierarchy on end, as shown in Exhibit 5.1. The CEO and senior administration form the narrow base that supports the rest of the organization. In the absence of this support, a Lean organization will collapse just as a man-made structure would. Senior leadership's role is to keep the organization focused, provide strategic direction, encourage employee involvement, and provide the resources necessary for execution of Lean.

The next level of the organizational hierarchy for Lean implementation is upper and middle management. Directors and managers are responsible for providing guidance to frontline staff, so they must develop a thorough understanding of Lean tools and principles. Every Lean implementation is different and presents new and sometimes complex situations. Directors and managers must develop the knowledge and experience necessary to deal with these different scenarios and ensure successful outcomes. This level of knowledge and experience is acquired over time through training and departmental application and, eventually, by leading kaizen events.

At the top of the organizational hierarchy for Lean implementation is frontline staff. These individuals are closest to the daily operations of the business and will have to internalize and live with

Exhibit 5.1: The Lean Organizational Hierarchy

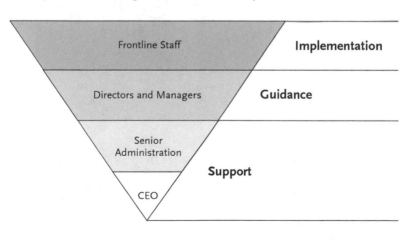

the changes. For this reason, it is logical that they be the ones to implement the changes.

CLOSING THE LAUNCH

The launch should conclude with a sincere appeal for staff participation. Close the launch with a question-and-answer period, and inform everyone present that training will be provided at a level appropriate for each individual's job responsibilities.

Subsequent meetings should be scheduled on a regular basis, preferably quarterly, to update the staff on the organization's progress, provide a venue for departments to present results from their implementation efforts, and give staff an opportunity to air their concerns and ask questions.

SUMMARY: A Properly Planned Launch

- A properly planned and implemented launch prepares the staff for what is to follow, thereby minimizing resistance, surprises, and the circulation of assumptions and rumors.

- The prospect of eliminating barriers to providing high-quality patient care is an ideal platform from which to launch a Lean transformation.

- It is important to make crystal clear that Lean targets wasteful processes and not people.

- A successful Lean transformation necessitates top-down commitment and bottom-up implementation.

CHAPTER 6

Appropriate Training

What is clear to you, is clear to you.

—Unknown

Training is the most essential element of cultural development. An organization's culture consists of beliefs, values, and attitudes based on the staff's work experiences. It is the way people see and do their jobs. Staff cannot be expected to embrace a new culture until they know what it will entail. How will their jobs change? What will they be expected to do differently? For what will they be held accountable? What will they need to learn? What is Lean, and what are its underlying principles? These questions must be answered before implementation begins.

Training should be commensurate with the three levels defined by the Lean organizational hierarchy depicted in Exhibit 5.1: support, guidance, and implementation. Support function training should focus on providing strategic direction, encouraging employee involvement, and keeping the organization focused. Guidance function training must generate a thorough understanding of Lean tools and concepts so that participants are able to coach staff members. Implementation function training should focus on identifying waste and actions that need to be taken to eliminate that waste.

SUPPORT FUNCTION TRAINING

The CEO and all of his direct reports should participate in support function training. Senior-level management need to know the "what" and "why" of Lean but not necessarily the "how": They must be able to speak the language of Lean and understand the principles, but they do not necessarily need to learn how to apply Lean tools.

The primary role of the support function is to provide strategic direction. The ability to provide strategic direction differentiates leadership from management. This responsibility encompasses much more than just creating a strategic plan. It includes strategic deployment (which is necessary to create vertical and horizontal alignment of the hospital's strategic objectives throughout the organization) and setting individual objectives relative to the hospital's areas of strategic focus. The support function also assigns accountability for these strategic goals and provides the resources necessary to achieve them. Finally, the support function keeps the organization focused. This job entails *genchi genbutsu*, Japanese for "go and see for yourself"—i.e., leaving the confines of one's office and becoming a visible presence in the organization's departments. Traditionally, the presence of a senior-level manager at the unit level indicated there was a problem or something was being done incorrectly. In a Lean organization, this presence is a welcome daily occurrence. The purpose of these visits is to demonstrate support, keep the organization focused, and aid in the development of a problem-solving culture. Therefore, support function training should advise senior management on how to conduct these visits. It should clarify that the role is a support function and not a "do what I say" function. Rather than fulfill the traditional managerial role of problem solver, leadership's goal in a Lean organization is to develop the staff's problem-solving skills. One way to do so is to ask pointed questions that engage staff and elicit their ideas. By developing frontline staff's problem-solving abilities, management creates a powerful dynamic for sustainable, repeatable success. All functions of the support role are essential to fostering a positive relationship of mutual trust and respect between leadership and staff.

GUIDANCE FUNCTION TRAINING

In a Lean organization the primary responsibility of directors and managers is to coach and develop their staff's problem-solving skills and to guide Lean implementation. They are mentors or *sensei*, the Japanese word for "teacher." Therefore, their training is the most comprehensive and does not end in the classroom.

Hospitals should schedule a multiday workshop to introduce Lean tools and principles to all directors and managers. The workshop should focus mainly on the use of Lean tools but also clearly define Lean principles and the concept of bottom-up implementation. Because people tend to want to apply Lean tools immediately, they neglect to discern the nature of the problem and its root cause. Consequently, they address only symptoms of the problem and thus leave the door wide open for the problem to resurface, sometimes with serious consequences. Workshop participants must learn that Lean tools are countermeasures to problems and that they must first understand the problem they are experiencing to be able to select the correct countermeasure.

The guidance function must internalize the three key Lean elements of standard work, user-friendliness, and unobstructed throughput and understand how Lean tools address these elements. Most important, directors and managers must learn to help their staff develop a heightened awareness for waste and then provide them with the resources they need to eliminate it.

Like the support function, the guidance function does not involve telling staff members what they have to do or how to do it. Rather, it involves developing the staff's problem-solving skills by asking pointed questions and engaging them in the problem-solving process. By repeatedly asking questions, mentors help staff arrive at a solution; in time, staff will pose these questions on their own.

IMPLEMENTATION FUNCTION TRAINING

Frontline staff decide the success or failure of a Lean initiative. They are the organization's process experts and most valuable asset. When these individuals are empowered to implement Lean, Lean culture flourishes.

Implementation function training best begins with a simple, unambiguous explanation of the state of healthcare in the United States and the need for change. Important points of emphasis include the cost of poor quality, the amount of waste in the healthcare system, and the need to work together for the good of the patient.

Although the definition of Lean (a system for the elimination of waste) may seem clear and simple enough, staff need to understand the definition of waste and that it is present in work processes, not in the people doing the work. Training can then teach staff to identify waste and actions necessary to eliminate it. These individuals are best equipped to identify waste because they continuously witness it in their daily activities.

Witnessing and recognizing are two different activities, however. To develop their ability to identify waste, staff have to change their perspective and no longer accept mistakes, inefficiencies, and other types of waste as circumstantial to the care delivery process. Training should demonstrate that even seemingly insignificant waste expends time and resources and has the potential to escalate problems and contribute to serious negative consequences. In some cases, simple fixes will suffice to eliminate identified waste; in others, more elaborate action will be necessary. In complex situations, staff should seek guidance from their directors or managers.

Do not assume that everyone has the same understanding of Lean or of their role in the initiative. Instill a common understanding of Lean throughout the organization.

SUMMARY: Appropriate Training

- Training is the most essential element of cultural development.

- Training should be commensurate with the three levels defined by the Lean organizational hierarchy: support, guidance, and implementation.

- The primary role of the support function is to provide strategic direction.

- In a Lean organization the primary responsibility of directors and managers is to coach and develop their staff.

- Frontline staff are the organization's process experts and its most valuable asset.

CHAPTER 7

Departmental Implementation

Tell me and I'll forget; show me and I may remember; involve me and I'll understand.

—Chinese proverb

Expertise with Lean tools cannot be acquired in a classroom. Although the objectives of developing standard work, user-friendliness, and unobstructed throughput are common to all Lean applications, the environment, regulatory requirements, scope, problems, and objectives involved in each situation are different. Because every possible scenario cannot be replicated in the classroom, this proficiency is attainable only through application of these tools in a real-world setting.

As soon as possible after training, workshop participants should apply the tools they have learned to use. It is important that these early applications be confined to participants' respective departments. At this stage, a multidisciplinary kaizen event that crosses departmental boundaries would be premature and could instigate boundary disputes. The department level presents many opportunities to apply Lean tools and principles, and only at this level do directors and managers have the authority to implement change.

By applying these tools and principles at the department level, staff are immersed in a learning environment and involved in the implementation process early on. Departmental implementation is also beneficial for the following reasons:

- The department becomes more efficient. Staff receive immediate positive feedback for their efforts, and the improvements lend credibility to the Lean initiative.
- Staff members are exposed to Lean tools and concepts in a familiar, comfortable environment.
- Directors and managers have an opportunity to gain experience and confidence in their guidance role.

Most important, application of Lean tools at the department level promotes a Lean culture. Management and staff learn together within the confines of their departments and internalize these concepts over time. When this internalization is complete, a Lean culture will prevail. The three elements supporting the House of Lean that are part of the culture-creating path—kaizen, jidoka, and respect for people (see exhibits 4.1 and 4.2)—become the status quo. In a culture of kaizen (continuous incremental improvement), staff are always looking for opportunities to improve. By engaging in jidoka (defined as "making problems obvious"), staff members recognize that only by reporting problems and implementing immediate problem resolution can the reoccurrence of these problems be eliminated. Respect for people (empowerment) is realized when the people who are doing the work and living with the changes are the same people implementing the improvements.

Departmental implementation does not need to be a formal, multiday kaizen event. Lean tools and concepts should be implemented over the course of the normal workday. In situations that demand a more methodical approach, implementation can follow the plan-do-check-act (PDCA) cycle.

THE PDCA CYCLE

Quality improvement experts such as W. Edwards Deming, Tai-ichi Ohno, Shigeo Shingo, Hiroyuki Hirano, and Joseph Juran introduced many tools in support of Lean concepts. The most famous of these tools, adopted by many healthcare organizations as their process improvement methodology, is Deming's PDCA cycle. Illustrated in Exhibit 7.1, the PDCA concept suggests that improvement is a cyclical process including the following steps:

- **Plan:** Identify a problem and develop a plan to solve it.
- **Do:** Implement the plan on a small scale.
- **Check:** Evaluate the results and compare them to the desired results.
- **Act:** Analyze the results and adopt, abandon, or alter the plan.

The cycle continues until the desired results are attained and the plan is adopted, at which point opportunities for additional

Exhibit 7.1: The Deming PDCA Cycle

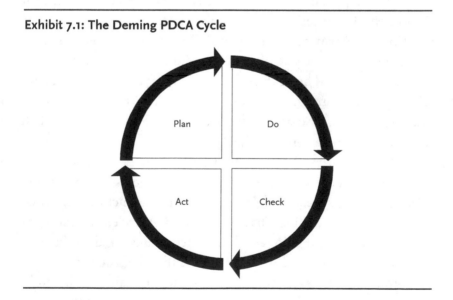

improvement are investigated and the cycle is revisited. Repeating the cycle constitutes continuous improvement.

Many hospitals and other healthcare providers have employed the PDCA cycle as a process improvement methodology for many years. Some of these organizations mistakenly believe that they must stop using the PDCA cycle if they decide to create a Lean enterprise. Almost all process improvement methodologies originated from Deming's model. It is a fundamental concept of continuous improvement and is the cycle employed during kaizen events.

THE A3 REPORT

Waste is not a product of physical processes only; it also is often abundant in abstract processes, such as reporting. Reports are typically compiled, bound, and tabbed in a book-like fashion. They are confusing, time-consuming to read and decipher, and often packed with extraneous information. The A3 report, developed by Toyota, was designed to eliminate this category of waste.

The A3 report is named after the size of the paper on which it is printed. According to international paper size standards, an 11″ × 17″ sheet of paper is designated as A3. Hence, A3 reports must be condensed to one side of an 11″ × 17″ sheet of paper. As a result, waste is eliminated on both ends; the report writer produces a concise document, and the task of reading the report is less laborious. The A3 report is also an excellent tool to use in developing staff members' problem-solving skills.

When folded in half, the A3 report becomes two standard 8.5″ × 11″ sheets of paper. If desired, two 8.5″ × 11″ sheets may be used in place of the A3 sheet. The left side of the report includes information about the planning phase of the PDCA cycle. On the right side, objectives of the do, check, and act phases are documented. This format obliges staff members to use the PDCA cycle, clarifies the problem, and helps staff determine the root cause of the problem so they may implement appropriate countermeasures.

Exhibit 7.2: Template for an A3 Problem-Solving Report

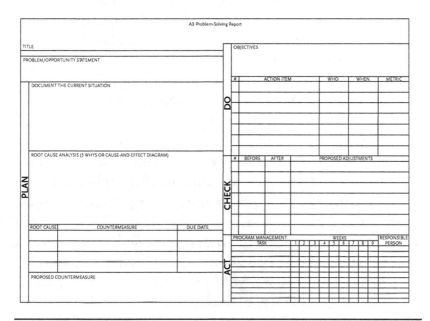

An example template for the A3 report is provided in Exhibit 7.2. Various other A3 report templates are also available for free download on the Internet. Once an organization selects a template, it should standardize all of its problem-solving reports to that template.

The left side of the form documents the plan for addressing the issue. After clearly stating the problem or opportunity to be addressed, the staff member observes and documents the process in question as it is being performed. Too often, this section is completed away from the action (e.g., in a meeting or at one's desk) and therefore depicts how the process is supposed to be conducted instead of how it is currently conducted. This documentation can include flowcharts, graphs, or drawings. The second section is reserved for a root cause analysis. The methods most commonly used to determine the root cause of a problem in Lean are the 5 Whys method and the cause-and-effect diagram. The planning phase concludes with a brainstorming session in which staff propose countermeasures for the identified root causes and select those that seem to be the best solutions to the problem. These measures should be written in the last section on the left side of the form along with an implementation deadline.

Documentation of the problem-solving process continues on the right side of the A3 report. The Do phase involves setting objectives and assigning action items. It is a test phase in which countermeasures should be implemented on a small scale to determine whether they are yielding the desired results. The Check phase entails comparing metrics taken before and after implementation of the countermeasures and making any necessary changes or adjustments. Once the desired level of improvement is achieved, the process enters the Act phase. The countermeasures are implemented on a full scale and the new standard work process is established.

An A3 report does not have to be completed for every problem encountered. The solutions to some problems are obvious and simple, and generation of an A3 report in such cases would only create more waste. Staff members who identify problems should turn to their directors and managers for guidance on how to proceed.

CONTINUOUS IMPROVEMENT STATUS BOARD

The purpose of departmental implementation is to teach staff to solve problems. They need to constantly question their processes, disclose problems, and make adjustments as needed rather than rationalize the methods they use to perform their duties. By implementing Lean tools on a daily basis, employees will internalize Lean concepts and the culture will slowly shift to one of continuous incremental improvement.

An excellent way to encourage improvement efforts is by tracking progress on a continuous improvement status board (see Exhibit 7.3). This board should be enlarged, laminated, and displayed in a central location. When staff members identify an area of waste,

No.	Problem/Issue/Opportunity	Countermeasure	Person Responsible	Date/Time Due	PDCA

CONTINUOUS IMPROVEMENT STATUS BOARD

ean Hospitals
Bringing Lean to Healthcare

they can write the problem and a proposed countermeasure on the board, along with their name.

Three rules regulate status board entries:

1. No one will be hired and no one will be fired. Hiring and firing are decisions for the department head and should not be proposed as a solution to a problem.
2. The organization will not purchase expensive equipment or software as a countermeasure. If a process is broken, the purchase of new software or equipment—such as an electronic medical record, a picture archiving and communication system (PACS), or a barcoding system—often increases the complexity of the problem.
3. The status board measure must be confined to the department head's area of influence so that staff members focus on what they can change rather than blame other departments for

their problems. Two departments can collaborate on an improvement effort, but at this stage no more than two departments should be involved.

When a staff member documents a problem on the status board, the department director or manager can meet with that individual to discuss the problem and the proposed countermeasure and advise him on how to proceed. As each phase of the PDCA cycle is completed, the corresponding section of the pie chart on the right side of the form is shaded to keep everyone informed about the status of a problem at a glance.

The continuous improvement status board should be a daily checkpoint of senior administrators' visits to hospital departments/units. They should discuss selected improvement efforts with the responsible staff member and review the A3 report. If the improvement effort has stalled, the senior-level manager can provide the guidance and support necessary to advance the initiative to the next level.

SHARING SUCCESSES

It is important to share successes with other departments and to recognize the staff's efforts. Quarterly assemblies should be scheduled for this purpose. Early on in the Lean transformation, it is advisable to schedule these assemblies monthly. Senior management should create a rotating schedule so that departments know in advance when they will be presenting their improvement efforts. The presentations should follow the A3 format and include photos or other documents to enhance the presentation. Members of senior administration need to be present at these assemblies to recognize and support staff efforts.

Departmental implementation encourages staff members to be active participants in the Lean transformation. This involvement promotes an understanding of Lean tools, ownership of problems, and pride in the organization's accomplishments. Before Lean principles can be internalized, they must be thoroughly understood, and this understanding is best acquired through guided application of Lean tools in a real-world setting.

SUMMARY: Departmental Implementation

- Departmental implementation is a key component in developing a Lean culture.

- The PDCA model is a fundamental concept of continuous improvement and is the cycle employed during kaizen events.

- Use of the A3 form obliges staff members to follow the PDCA cycle, understand the issue, and determine the root cause of a problem before implementing countermeasures.

- The purpose of departmental implementation is to teach staff to solve problems and to expose them to Lean tools and principles. Ultimately, the goal is to have them internalize these tools and principles and implement them within their departments on a daily basis.

CHAPTER 8

Jidoka, Kaizen, and Respect for People

Many hands make light work.

—John Heywood

The culture-creating path of the Lean implementation model concludes with the synthesis of three of the four elements supporting the House of Lean depicted in Exhibit 4.2: jidoka (making problems obvious), kaizen (continuous incremental improvement), and respect for people (empowerment). The House of Lean is a model of a Lean organization. As stated earlier, the durability of a Lean organization, as that of a house, is determined by the care and coordinated effort that went into its construction. Failure to properly implement the steps necessary to instill a Lean culture will result in an unstable transformation that is susceptible to outside forces and destined to collapse.

JIDOKA (MAKING PROBLEMS OBVIOUS)

Industrialist and inventor Sakichi Toyoda founded Toyoda Automatic Loom Works, Ltd., in 1926. In 1924 Sakichi invented an automatic power loom, his most famous invention. This loom operated at high speeds, could be kept running while shuttles were changed, and automatically stopped if a thread broke. Seemingly insignificant, this last feature eliminated defects, one of the seven categories of waste, through human intervention. When the machine stopped, the operator reattached the thread and restarted the machine, ensuring that all products coming off the looms were defect free. This principle later became known as jidoka, a key element of the Toyota Production System.

Jidoka literally translates to "automation with the human touch." However, the fundamental concept of jidoka is best defined as "making problems obvious." Many organizations in the United States find this concept counterintuitive. Department heads invariably want to distinguish their department from other departments in the organization. One way of doing so is to have a zero error rate. To achieve this objective, department heads sometimes conceal errors or discourage staff from reporting them. This practice is especially prevalent in organizations that have not properly deployed their strategic plan, thereby compelling department heads to assume a departmental focus. The Lean philosophy does just the opposite; it encourages staff to expose flaws in the system. If errors and potential errors are not reported, they cannot be fixed and will persist.

The benefits of reporting errors and taking immediate action to resolve problems are best illustrated by the success of the airline industry. On November 12, 2001, American Airlines flight 587 crashed in Belle Harbor, Queens, New York. On August 27, 2006, Comair flight 5191 crashed during a routine takeoff at Blue Grass Airport in Lexington, Kentucky. These two crashes mark the beginning and the end of what has been hailed the safest period in commercial aviation history in the United States. For almost five years, the commercial airline industry in the United States experienced zero passenger deaths (KLTV 2006).

This incredible safety record has been attributed to the implementation of the Aviation Safety Reporting System (ASRS). Pilots, dispatchers, airport personnel, air traffic controllers, mechanics, baggage handlers, and cabin crew are encouraged to report problems or potential problems that might jeopardize passenger or crew safety. These detailed reports include the time, date, and location of the issue; the type of aircraft and the roles of the people involved; the factors contributing to the problem; and a narrative section featuring an assessment and a synopsis of the situation. Anyone can view these reports online at http://asrs.nasa.gov. The ASRS investigates every report in a timely manner and takes appropriate action to correct the problem. To the system's credit, it takes corrective action not only on the aircraft for which the report was generated but on all aircraft of the same type across the industry. For example, if American Airlines reports a problem with a Boeing 737, all airline companies are notified of the issue and required to fix the anomaly on all Boeing 737s in service.

Error Reporting

When we discover a mistake or defect, our first inclination is to find someone to blame. This reaction is human nature. Most people grow up accustomed to this behavior, so it has become an instinctive reaction anytime something goes wrong. At home, in school, and at work, we learn that we will be absolved of a mistake and will not be penalized if we find someone else to blame for it. This phenomenon was illustrated in a recently aired television commercial featuring a group of senior leaders sitting around a table in a boardroom. The leader is soliciting suggestions for a solution to a serious problem confronting the organization. Silence prevails. Feeling pressured to deliver on his boss's request, a member of the team suggests they conduct a "blame-storming session." He points his finger at the woman sitting across the table from him and proclaims, "I blame Ellen."

The humor in this commercial is an exaggeration of real life. Few people would blatantly point a finger at someone and blame her for a problem. Blame is more commonly established behind closed doors or disguised as an effort to determine the root cause of the problem (e.g., "Who was the last one to use this machine?").

The fear of blame is the primary deterrent to error reporting. Regardless of why or how blame is assigned, people associate it with enormous consequences. Studies suggest that as few as 1.5 percent of all adverse events in hospitals are reported (Shojania et al. 2001). If errors are not reported, their causes persist, permitting the errors to reoccur, possibly with more serious consequences.

The failure to report errors is a serious problem in healthcare. An even more serious issue is the belief that a problem can be solved by blaming, reprimanding, or terminating the person who made the mistake. Although people make mistakes, the causes of the mistakes are generally rooted in complex or inadequate systems. For this reason, blaming is futile. Blame and the reprimands and disciplinary action associated with it contribute nothing to the reduction or elimination of errors. Instead these actions hurt morale, increase anxiety among staff, humiliate those who have been singled out, and ultimately undermine patient care.

Another obstacle to error reporting is management's failure to take immediate action to address the root cause of the problem. This failure to act is inconsistent with Lean principles, and staff will perceive managers who procrastinate as insincere about the Lean initiative. Error reporting is a difficult undertaking for healthcare professionals (or anyone, for that matter), especially when the error resulted from one's own actions. No one wants to admit to a mistake, even if there is no threat of blame. People's self-imposed standards and the feelings of incompetence that result when they do not meet those standards often prevent them from reporting errors. To overcome these convictions, they must recognize that by reporting errors they are acting in the best interest of their patients, the organization, and their fellow workers, and they must witness the corrective action taken in response to their report. Some organizations have an error-reporting hotline that connects callers to voice mail, but this method does not instill confidence that someone is listening and will address the problem. A machine cannot ask clarifying questions, gain a full understanding and appreciation of the problem, take corrective action, or offer reassurance. For these reasons, the reporting method must involve interaction with another person.

All staff must know what action they should take if they make a mistake or witness a situation that jeopardizes patient safety. When an error is reported, the appropriate reaction should be one of gratitude for the courage and benevolence demonstrated by the staff member making the report. Management should never express annoyance or disappointment about the error or any person who contributed to it. The slightest demonstration of negativity could prevent staff from reporting future mistakes.

Equally important is for staff to report potential errors, commonly referred to as *near misses*. Potential errors are conditions that could cause a defect but are intercepted before they do. For example, if a nurse discovers and correctly re-files the medical records of two patients that had been switched because they have the same last name, this event would be considered a near miss. Had the nurse not discovered the discrepancy and corrected it, a serious or even lethal error could have occurred. Such situations normally would not be reported as an error, and consequently the system flaw would not be addressed and the impending error and related consequences would remain a threat to patient safety. Obviously, it is preferable to address a potential error than to wait until it is manifested to address it. In addition, people are less likely to feel the need to blame someone when reporting potential errors. Instead, such discoveries often provoke a sense of worth and competence in the detector. This reaction is appropriate; in most situations, people who spot a potential error want others to know about it. Hence, people are more likely to report potential errors and participate in correcting the process anomaly that caused them.

Cultivation of a blameless environment in which people feel comfortable reporting errors and potential errors precedes the development of a Lean culture. Fundamental to Lean principles are (1) a focus on the process anomaly rather than on the individual who made the error and (2) immediate initiative to address the root cause of the problem.

KAIZEN (CONTINUOUS INCREMENTAL IMPROVEMENT)

The relentless bombings of Japan by the Allied forces and the atomic bombing of Hiroshima and Nagasaki at the end of World War II left the country devastated. Japan had to rebuild its entire infrastructure, literally from the ground up. Doing so required that the country continuously improve to meet the challenges of the day. As a result, continuous improvement became a necessary component of the personal, social, and work life of the Japanese people.

Kaizen (pronounced *kī'zen*) has been described as the single most important element contributing to the success of the Toyota Production System. The term is derived from two Japanese words—*kai*, which means "change," and *zen*, meaning "for the better." Hence, kaizen translates to "change for the better" or "improvement." However, the concept of kaizen relates more precisely to ongoing or continuous improvement. Kaizen involves everyone in the organization—senior leaders, directors, managers, and staff—and is deeply ingrained in the Lean culture.

In his book *Kaizen: The Key to Japan's Competitive Success*, Masaaki Imai (1986) suggests that business management has two major components: maintenance and improvement. Responsibilities for these components are allocated to four distinct levels in an organization: senior leadership, directors, managers, and staff. In the context of his book, *maintenance* means conducting business in accordance with the policies and procedures established by an organization's leaders. Accordingly, the majority of the maintenance component falls on staff members because they conduct the daily operations of the business. The higher one is in the organizational hierarchy, the lesser one's responsibility for maintenance. *Improvement* means refining policies and procedures and thereby enhancing the products or services offered by the enterprise. Appropriately, the majority of the responsibility for improvement is allocated to senior leadership and lessens as job functions approach daily business operations. Imai suggests that most organizations interpret improvement as radical innovative change, or *kaikaku*, and therefore a cavernous void exists between maintenance and innovation because most organizations fail to take advantage of opportunities for small incremental change. Furthermore, in the absence of an internal drive for improvement, external forces such as competition or market conditions can force change on the organization.

In a Lean organization, kaizen fills this gap. The responsibility for kaizen is evenly distributed to all levels of the organization. Everyday collaboration to improve the care delivery system is the essence of Lean culture in a healthcare organization. For improvement to be sustained, maintenance and improvement must become inseparable.

When someone takes on a new position, that person spends much of his time learning the policies and procedures established by the organization. With time, the person becomes more proficient in his duties and begins to question why things are done a certain way. In turn, these questions provoke ideas for improvement. Many organizations either ignore such ideas or postpone their consideration and eventually forget them. This missed opportunity to implement employee suggestions is a major source of waste. Furthermore, inaction discourages staff from voicing their ideas and promotes indifference. Conversely, kaizen encourages employee suggestions and their application.

RESPECT FOR PEOPLE (EMPOWERMENT)

Every Toyota manufacturing plant runs a yellow cord, called an *andon cord*, parallel to the assembly line (*andon* is the Japanese word for "light"). This cord hangs within easy reach of the assembly line workers and is used to alert supervisors that a problem has been spotted and needs attention. When a worker pulls the cord, a section of a large board lights up, indicating the worker's location along the assembly line. If the worker cannot solve the problem on his own, he pulls the cord a second time, which halts production. Immediately, supervisors or engineers proceed to the location indicated on the board to assist the worker. Giving an assembly line worker the authority to stop the assembly line was unheard of in American manufacturing plants, whereas at Toyota, workers have that authority and are expected to use it if they cannot resolve a problem, even a minor one. This concept is called "respect for people" and is a supporting element of the Toyota Production System.

Contrary to what many people think, respect for people in a Lean culture does not simply constitute patting staff members on the back and extolling their accomplishments. Rather, such actions are gestures that managers extend as a result of having respect for people. In a Lean culture, respect for people means acknowledging that all people are experts at what they do. Whether their job involves neurosurgery or cleaning a patient's room, they know the best way to do the job, what does and does not work, and the problems associated with the job, and they usually can offer sound recommendations on how to fix these problems or improve the job's processes. Accordingly, management should solicit staff members' input regarding problems, mistakes, and inefficiencies affecting their duties. By encouraging their input, management demonstrates respect for their knowledge and abilities.

Too often improvement initiatives are conducted behind closed doors without the involvement of the staff members who do the work. The Lean philosophy encourages everyone associated with the faulty process to help develop a solution. Toyota managers involve staff in the problem-solving process by asking employees to define the problem, identify the cause of the problem, suggest solutions for eliminating the problem, and demonstrate that their proposal would ensure the problem will not return. Employees are then tasked with implementing their proposed solutions (Womack 2008). Throughout this process, management engages employees in dialogue to ensure they have identified the root cause of the problem, supports their efforts, and provides the resources and guidance they need to resolve the problem successfully. In this type of environment, staff become more confident and able to make bigger decisions on their own, and the pleasure and gratification they experience as a result of their contribution to the resolution encourage them to identify other problem-solving opportunities.

Respect for people is mutual. Management demonstrates this respect by encouraging the involvement of staff members. In return, staff members demonstrate respect by recognizing that improvement is not possible without management's support and guidance.

In most organizations, including hospitals, the customary method of addressing problems is to assign responsibility for problem resolution to a team of "quality experts." In many cases these individuals have no experience with the affected process. They hold regular meetings to discuss causes and solutions to several problems plaguing the organization and typically prioritize them according to the problems' visibility or, more specifically, administration's desire to resolve them. Consequently, lower priority problems fall to the bottom of the list, where they may remain unresolved for months, for years, or indefinitely. This approach to problem resolution conflicts with the concept of kaizen and constitutes waste in the form of missed opportunities.

Many times these quality teams fail to address the root cause of the problem and propose workarounds or stopgap measures that add work to an already cumbersome process. For example, implementing checks and double checks only increases the workload of an already overburdened staff. A quality team is not acting incompetently by resorting to such measures, however. It is likely overwhelmed with a long list of problems and is undoubtedly experiencing intense pressure to develop solutions. Feeling compelled to deal with these problems as expeditiously as possible, team members are unable to use their expert problem-solving skills to their fullest extent.

In the early 1990s many buzzwords infiltrated corporate America. Company presentations and business documents were rife with such terms as *leverage, proactive, paradigm*, and *synergy*.

The word *empowerment* was also popular. However, as is the case with all buzzwords, the meaning of empowerment was open to interpretation. To empower someone means granting that person authority. When the limits of that authority are not clearly defined, empowerment can be a dangerous dispensation. Consequently, many organizational leaders witnessed the havoc that resulted from the ill-considered application of empowerment, and managers and supervisors shuddered at the thought of relinquishing their authority, fearful that their employers would no longer value their services. These events and perceptions left an indelible mark on the concept of empowerment in the minds of many organizational leaders.

Creation of a Lean enterprise is an enormous and incessantly demanding task that will not come to fruition without the collaboration and enthusiasm of all hospital staff. Accordingly, an organization must dispel any negativity about the concept of empowerment lingering from past experiences. When leaders encourage empowerment, employees see their work processes with new eyes. They question inconsistencies and look for opportunities to improve. The concept of empowerment also harmonizes with the concepts of jidoka and kaizen. When granted and defined properly, empowerment can save time, money, and most important, lives.

The introduction of the Toyota Creative Idea Suggestion System by Toyota management in 1951 illustrates the improvement potential of the Lean elements discussed in this chapter. In 1988 Toyota marked the receipt of its twenty-millionth suggestion from staff (Yasuda 1991). In the last decade, the system has generated more than 2 million ideas annually, lifting its lifetime total to more than 40 million suggestions. Even more impressive is Toyota's 90 percent implementation rate (Vasishtha 2011).

SUMMARY: JIDOKA, KAIZEN, AND RESPECT FOR PEOPLE

- The culture-creating path of the Lean implementation model concludes with the synthesis of jidoka (making problems obvious), kaizen (continuous incremental improvement), and respect for people (empowerment).

- Cultivation of a blameless environment in which people feel comfortable reporting errors and potential errors precedes the development of a Lean environment.

- For improvement to be sustained, maintenance and improvement must become inseparable.

- The concept of respect for people generates a sense of problem ownership and is consistent with the concepts of jidoka and kaizen.

SECTION 3

SYSTEMS THINKING

CHAPTER 9

The System-Creating Path

Discontent is the first necessity of progress.

—Thomas Edison

To achieve a Lean transformation, an organization must function as a system. *Lean* is defined as "a system for the absolute elimination of waste," and *system* is defined as "a set of correlated members forming a unitary whole" (Ohno 1988; Dictionary.com 2011). Departmental boundaries must come down so that all hospital functions focus on the patient and the patient's needs.

Exhibit 9.1 illustrates the system-creating path of the Lean implementation model. This path is extremely difficult to navigate because it has been forged over years or even decades of doing things the way they have always been done. Staff members do not want to change even though intuitively they know that change is necessary. People are comfortable in their jobs; they know all the ins and outs, and this knowledge affords a sense of security. Change almost always involves having to learn something new, and this prospect often induces an unfounded sense of anxiety in many staff members. Furthermore, the idea of change provokes fear—fear of losing one's identity, fear of failure, fear of success, and fear of leaving one's comfort zone. Staff may not be happy with their processes—they may complain about them and even endure hardships because of them—but in their minds the status quo is better than change.

Exhibit 9.1: The System-Creating Path of the Lean Implementation Model

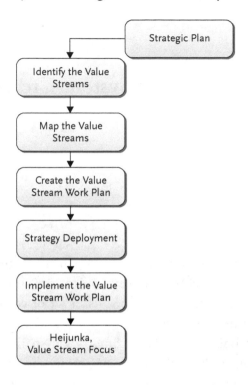

People are inclined to tolerate adverse circumstances to which they are accustomed rather than put forth the effort—and experience the discomfort and apprehension—involved in changing those circumstances. But they will reach a point at which they can no longer tolerate adverse situations left unchanged, and change must and will ensue.

The present care delivery system has been left unchanged for centuries. In an article titled, "Healthcare's Need for Revolutionary Change," Dr. Martin Merry (2003) suggests that the healthcare industry is "built essentially around a craft model rooted not in the 20th or even the 19th century, but in the 18th century." Changes to this complex and outdated system are long overdue.

THE NEED FOR CHANGE

As patients, we assume that the healthcare we receive is high quality and that our caregivers will take every precaution to minimize the spread of infection, yet the Centers for Disease Control and Prevention estimates that annually approximately 2 million patients contract a nosocomial infection (i.e., an infection patients acquire during their stay in a hospital) (CDC 2000). (Conservative estimates of the rate of mortality resulting from nosocomial infections are as high as 70,000 deaths annually [CDC 2000].) We assume that the medication we are prescribed is correct and that it is administered in the correct dosage, yet the US Food and Drug Administration estimates that at least one person dies every day and another 1.3 million people are injured each year as a result of medication errors (FDA 2009). We assume that our surgery will proceed safely and without incident, yet surgical errors account for thousands of injuries and deaths every year in the United States. A study published in *Health Services Research* found that one out of every ten patients who died within 90 days of surgery did so because of a preventable error (Encinosa and Hellinger 2008; AHRQ 2008). Surgeries in US hospitals have been performed on the wrong arm, leg, eye, kidney, breast, lung, and almost any other body part that has a duplicate, and even on the wrong patient. We assume that the hospital will provide safe, effective, and equitable medical care as efficiently as possible and that we will leave the hospital healthy or on the road to recovery (IOM 2001). But we assume wrongly. Quality in healthcare is, in reality, mediocre. The quality statistics associated with hospitals and healthcare organizations in the United States are so poor that similar statistics in any other industry would not be tolerated. For obvious reasons, anything less than perfect quality should not and cannot be tolerated in healthcare.

The staggering financial ramifications resulting from poor quality in healthcare are another impetus for change. The estimated annual cost of poor quality and waste in healthcare in the United States is more than $1 trillion (National Coalition on Health Care 2010). More specifically, this cost is attributed to mishaps such as medical errors, duplicate and unnecessary tests, medication errors, hospital-acquired infections, repeat procedures, increased hospitalization due to patients not receiving recommended care, inefficient processes, and more. David Lawrence, retired chairman and CEO of the Kaiser Foundation Health Plan, summarized these categories of waste as "overuse, underuse, misuse, duplication, system failures, unnecessary repetition, poor communication, and inefficiency" (Reid et al. 2005).

The nonmonetary consequences of poor quality and waste in healthcare are even worse. The IOM report *To Err Is Human* (2000) estimated that as many as 98,000 people die annually as a result of medical errors that could have been prevented and that more than one million patients are injured annually.

In a 2007 *CBS News* interview, Donald Berwick, then president and CEO of the Institute for Healthcare Improvement and later administrator of the Centers for Medicare & Medicaid Services, described hospitals as "very audacious places still generally run on outdated systems." Later in the interview he went on to describe hospitals as "very dangerous places." His comments were not meant to create fear among the public or to cause people to be horrified by the prospect of going to the hospital but rather to bring to light the dire need to change the care delivery system.

These conditions are not the result of incompetence or apathy on the part of healthcare professionals. These individuals are highly trained, experienced, caring people who want to do what is best for their patients. However, the current care delivery system in hospitals does not support their efforts. Decades of working around problems, implementing stopgap measures, and failing to acknowledge the need for change in care delivery have all contributed to an extremely complex and outmoded care delivery system. So many layers of work have been added to existing processes and handed down to new staff members over the years that the present staff cannot explain why processes are carried out the way they are. Their rationale commonly amounts to "That's the way we've always done it." As a result, the present care delivery system is made up of complicated, flawed processes that allow errors to occur and fosters a culture that is not centered on patients and their needs. How it happened, however, is far less important than the answer to the question "What are we going to do about it?"

The majority of hospital administrators, doctors, nurses, technologists, and other hospital staff members are aware of the problems with the care delivery system. When presented with statistical data indicating its inadequacies, they demonstrate little if any surprise. Instead these data raise a few eyebrows, solicit some disheartened headshakes, or invoke a barely audible expression of disappointment. These reactions are not a display of indifference on the part of these individuals, however. On the contrary, they are extremely concerned, but they are not surprised. Such statistics are almost expected and are viewed as unfortunate ramifications intrinsic to the system. The first decisive step toward system improvement is to cease to accept poor quality and waste as inherent. Unless we become discontented with the current healthcare delivery process, we won't take steps to improve it, and it will deteriorate even further. Present statistics will pale in comparison to those in the future if change does not occur. Healthcare can no longer maintain the status quo.

The phrase "survival of the fittest," coined by Charles Darwin, summons visions of the biggest and strongest species thriving and reproducing in their environment. However, natural selection is not directly proportional to size and strength but to the ability of a species to adapt to an ever-changing environment. The same is true of healthcare organizations. An organization's size and power do not make it more likely to survive tough times or grow. To thrive, an organization must adapt its care delivery system to the changing healthcare environment.

QUALITY VERSUS FINANCIAL FOCUS

During turbulent economic times, hospital leaders instinctively direct their attention to stabilizing finances. Dwindling reimbursements, the increasing cost of supplies and pharmaceuticals, the shortage of healthcare workers, changing technology, and loss of revenue to physician-owned outpatient clinics place intense pressure on hospital leaders to make quick decisions and produce timely and measureable results. Budgets are cut, spending is scrutinized, programs are put on hold, equipment purchases are deferred, and staff reductions ensue. These reactive strategies, which permeate most healthcare organizations, appear sound and logical, but in reality they incite mishaps that create more work, bigger problems, and widespread disorder. Instead of improving the situation, leaders' impulsive decisions often provoke greater financial instability in the form of higher costs, lost revenue, and missed opportunities.

These habitual responses to financial instability have a significant common characteristic: They neglect quality, not intentionally, but indirectly. A hospital cannot provide high-quality care and services without the necessary resources of time, money, and staff. Often hospital leaders' reactive responses to financial stress inadvertently lessen the availability of these resources and thus indirectly diminish the quality of care.

That is not to say that quality is ignored. The desire to provide quality care for patients is an inherent characteristic of almost every healthcare provider. Instead, they put quality on hold until the funds, time, and people are available to address the quality issue and implement work-arounds that create more work, add to the complexity of the care delivery process, and introduce additional quality issues, often of a more serious nature. For example, a nurse consults her hospital's prescription dispensing system and finds that her medication orders have not yet been delivered to her unit. She discovers that by entering all of her standard medication orders as STAT (i.e., urgent) orders, she can ensure timely delivery to the unit. However, this misrepresentation requires the pharmacist to work harder and faster to fulfill these orders in addition to fulfilling an already lengthy list of true STAT orders, which in turn makes him prone to commit errors and may delay the delivery of medications to a patient in genuine need. Work-arounds often masquerade as solutions, thereby eradicating the urgency to correct the root cause of the problem. Consequently, the problem is never formally and correctly resolved.

Healthcare organizations often address quality problems after receiving a complaint from patients or patients' family members. Again, this approach to improvement is reactive. Professor Noriaki Kano illustrated the futility of reacting to customer complaints in his Kano Model, shown in Exhibit 9.2. Kano identified three attributes of products and services that affect customer satisfaction. The first he called *dis-satisfiers*. Dis-satisfiers are features of a product or service that a customer expects. If they are not provided, the customer will complain. Dis-satisfiers never cross the horizontal axis of the Kano Model and therefore never generate customer satisfaction.

The second of these attributes he called *satisfiers*. Satisfiers are the same as dis-satisfiers except they do not provoke customer complaints. Instead, the customer will ask for the satisfier (i.e., feature or performance effort) if it is lacking or missing. Customer satisfaction is low when satisfiers are low or deficient; conversely, customer satisfaction is high when satisfiers are high or substantial. This attribute is linear, meaning that the level of customer satisfaction is directly proportional to the intensity of the performance effort or plenitude of the feature.

The last attribute is called *delighters*. Delighters are unexpected benefits that enhance the customer's experience. The delighter vector never dips below the horizontal axis, indicating that delighters can only increase customer satisfaction if they are provided but will never cause dissatisfaction if they are not provided. Exhibit 9.2 shows that the level of customer satisfaction can never rise above

Exhibit 9.2: The Kano Model for Customer Satisfaction

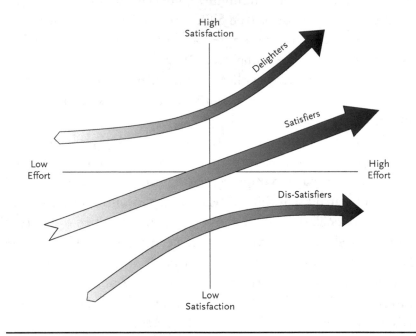

the horizontal axis if an organization just reacts to customer complaints (dis-satisfiers). In other words, its customers will never be more than "not dissatisfied." Hospitals need to put an end to reacting only to patient complaints and create a care delivery process that consistently satisfies and often delights their patients.

The biggest disincentive to adopting a quality focus is its delayed effect on an organization's finances. Quality is a cost avoidance measure, but an anticipatory effort to eliminate errors that may or may not occur is unlikely to be viewed as such. For example, a quality initiative associated with reducing ventilator-acquired pneumonia (VAP) may provide impressive results from a quality standpoint, but because hospitals do not budget for the treatment of VAP patients, any positive results appearing on the organization's financial statement as a result of the quality initiative will not be attributed to those efforts. Any correlation between quality and financial results is further masked by the amount of time it takes for savings realized from quality improvement projects to materialize on the organization's financial statement; it is not uncommon for quality improvement efforts to take six months to a year to produce measureable results.

In contrast, financial improvement efforts produce immediate, measurable, and seemingly impressive results. If budgeted new equipment is not purchased, if improvement programs are not funded, or if the workforce is reduced, the results are immediately apparent on the organization's financial statements. The pressures on hospital leaders subsequently subside, and they are often praised for taking on a difficult and unpopular task. Unfortunately, this approach is short-sighted and will lead to greater financial instability.

The most effective method for eliminating the stresses and strains that accompany financial frailty is to minimize the probability of a volatile financial state. The only way of going about this task is to establish a quality focus. Aristotle said, "Quality is not an act, it is a habit." Hospitals must instill in their staffs the habit of providing the highest-quality care possible for their patients. Every one of us wants and expects no less when we enter a hospital. The IOM report *Crossing the Quality Chasm: A New Health System for the 21st Century* (2001) indicates that "Fundamental reform of health care is needed to ensure that all Americans receive care that is safe, effective, patient centered, timely, efficient, and equitable." This statement describes the kind of healthcare a Lean hospital delivers. In a Lean organization, the certainty that a quality focus will promote financial stability is universally shared.

SUMMARY: The System-Creating Path

- People are more inclined to tolerate adverse circumstances to which they are accustomed than to put forth the effort and experience the discomfort and apprehension involved in changing those circumstances.

- People will reach a point at which they can no longer tolerate adverse situations left unchanged, and change must and will ensue. The present care delivery system has been left unchanged for centuries.

- Healthcare can no longer maintain the status quo. The care delivery process must change.

- The primary focus in changing the care delivery system must be the patient and the patient's needs.

CHAPTER 10

Identify the Value Streams

Efforts and courage are not enough without purpose and direction.
—John F. Kennedy

Leaders often fail to appreciate the level of effort required to transform an organization, and as a result they attempt to implement improvement efforts across the entire hospital. When everything is a priority, nothing is a priority, and little gets accomplished. As described in Chapter 1, the most typical implementation scenario is to schedule and conduct a series of kaizen events targeted at solving problems. Often after a year or two, these events fail to produce the improvement, cost reduction, and growth expected, and the Lean initiative falls by the wayside. Lean is cataloged along with other failed attempts at transformation, and the organization's leaders search for the newest solutions to organizational ineffectiveness. They do not recognize that no approach to achieving greater organizational effectiveness can be accomplished in one fell swoop.

To escape this cycle of failure, senior leaders must focus improvement efforts on specific areas. Lean methodology calls these areas *value streams*. Focusing improvement efforts on value streams does not preclude other improvement efforts, but the value streams should be the focus of the organization's large-scale improvement efforts.

THE VALUE STREAM DEFINED

The first step in the system-creating path of the Lean implementation model is to identify the value streams. A value stream encompasses all the processes necessary to provide a product or service. Value streams usually cross departmental boundaries, so improvement efforts are necessarily collaborative. In contrast to a process, the value stream includes all departments involved in delivering value to the patient.

In their book *Lean Thinking*, James Womack and Daniel Jones (1996) define the value stream as:

> [T]he set of all the specific actions required to bring a specific product through the three critical management tasks of any business: *the problem-solving task* running from concept through detailed design and engineering to production launch, the *information management task* running from order-taking through detailed scheduling to delivery, and the *physical transformation task* proceeding from raw materials to a finished product in the hands of the customer.

Although this definition is detailed and comprehensive, it could be confusing and difficult to apply to the healthcare environment. To make the three critical management tasks included in the definition more relevant to healthcare, we first have to recognize that healthcare has two value streams: the patient value stream and the product value stream.

Patient Value Streams

On the patient side, we redefine the three management tasks as follows:

- *The admission task* runs from patient presentation through registration to patient assessment.

- *The service task* runs from diagnostic testing or procedures to assessment of test results and care planning.
- *The discharge task* runs from care delivery through patient monitoring to patient discharge.

In the context of an inpatient admission through the emergency department (ED), for example, each task in this value stream might comprise the following elements:

- *The admission task:* presentation, registration, triage, and ED nurse/physician assessment
- *The service task:* collection of specimens, laboratory tests and diagnostic imaging, receipt of the laboratory test results, radiologist's report to the ED, and diagnosis and issuance of treatment orders by ED physician
- *The discharge task:* provision of any immediate treatment required, bed assignment, confirmation of the need to admit the patient by the hospitalist or attending physician, notification of availability of assigned bed, ED nurse's report to the inpatient unit, transport arrangements, room preparation, delivery of medications, additional testing, provision of care in the inpatient unit, and patient discharge

As this breakdown illustrates, the process requires a collaborative effort of several departments, including the ED, laboratory services, diagnostic imaging, transport, environmental services, the admitting office, the pharmacy, the inpatient unit, and case management.

Product Value Streams

On the product side, we redefine the three management tasks as follows:

- *The input task* runs from placement of the order for product components with vendors through receipt of the ordered product components.
- *The processing task* runs from receipt of physician orders through collection of product components to product processing.
- *The output task* runs from documentation and verification of results through delivery of a finished product to the customer.

For example, the tasks included in the value stream for processing blood specimens by laboratory services could be broken down into the following elements:

- *The input task:* issuance of purchase orders for supplies, such as specimen collection devices, reagents, and petri dishes, and receipt of these supplies
- *The processing task:* verification of physician orders and collection and processing of specimens
- *The output task*: documentation and verification of test results and delivery of test results to physician for diagnosis

These examples demonstrate the complexity of the value stream. Mapping all the value streams in a hospital would be a daunting task. Therefore, senior leaders have to identify which value streams they need to focus on to achieve their short-term strategic goals.

IDENTIFYING THE VALUE STREAMS

Strategic plans typically address several areas of strategic focus, such as quality, finance, cultivation of a rewarding work environment, and patient satisfaction. The strategic objectives associated with these areas are usually general. For example, a strategic objective for quality might be "to establish consistent delivery of care that demonstrates excellence in clinical quality and patient safety." Similarly, a strategic objective for finance could be "to implement revenue enhancement measures and enact cost containment measures to nurture long-term fiscal stability." The generality of these objectives could encompass every value stream imaginable in the organization. To be able to identify specific value streams, leaders must delve deeper into the strategic initiative to identify what actions the hospital would need to take to demonstrate excellence in clinical care, enhance revenue, or contain cost. Objectives should be crafted to reflect the SMART acronym, meaning they should be specific, measureable, attainable, relevant, and time bound.

For example, a SMART objective for finance might be "to enact cost containment measures by the end of the fiscal year to reduce bottom line expenses by 15 percent over last year's expenses." This goal is specific, measureable (i.e., a reduction of 15 percent), attainable, relevant, and time bound (i.e., by the end of the fiscal year). However, to identify the value streams targeted by this objective, leaders must delve even deeper and define the specific tasks that must be carried out to achieve the SMART objective. An action item might be "to enact cost containment measures in the pharmacy to reduce the costs associated with obtaining, preparing, and dispensing inpatient medications by 25 percent by the end of the third quarter." This action item identifies the pharmacy as a value stream on which to focus.

The pharmacy value stream could be defined as follows:

- *The input task* includes ordering and receipt of medications and supplies.
- *The processing task* includes receipt of inpatient medication orders prescribed by physicians, preparation of medications, and batch order processing of existing prescriptions.

- *The output task* includes verification of preparation and delivery of medications to customers.

This breakdown may appear to be a simplified definition of what a pharmacy does, but the objective at this point is just to identify the value stream—that is, to identify the targeted area (the pharmacy) and the scope of that focus (from ordering supplies to delivering medications for inpatients).

Each value stream involves many departments, and therefore much coordinated effort is required to accomplish SMART objectives. For example, the pharmacy might work with the purchasing department to reduce the costs of supplies and pharmaceuticals, work with the inpatient units to prevent preparation of duplicate and discontinued medications and ensure timely and accurate delivery of medications, and so on. Aside from the purchasing department, the pharmacy's value stream might include outside suppliers, the ED, surgical services, and diagnostic imaging.

As mentioned earlier, because of the level of effort necessary to achieve the strategic objectives for each value stream, leaders are advised to identify only a few value streams to work on each year. Each identified value stream will require much effort and collaboration to achieve the desired future state. If too many value streams are identified, tasks will overlap and staff will become overwhelmed, confused, and discouraged. Three is a reasonable number of value streams to identify in a fiscal year. While a focus on three value streams might seem too small of an effort to have an impact on the organization, more than three could easily prove to be too many if each of the three value streams chosen has an extensive scope.

Attempts to meet ambiguous strategic objectives leave department directors and managers overwhelmed. By focusing improvement efforts on the value streams that contribute most to the advancement of strategic initiatives, senior administrators provide direction and consolidate efforts. Focused effort in one value stream benefits not only the department at the heart of the value stream but also all other departments that interact with that value stream. For example, improvement efforts in the pharmacy value stream identified earlier will help the purchasing department acquire a better understanding of the pharmacy's needs and make more educated purchases, thereby reducing costs. Ultimately, the patient and the organization as a whole benefit from these improvements.

SUMMARY: Identify the Value Streams

- Value streams encompass all the processes necessary to provide a product or service.

- Senior leaders must identify which value streams they need to focus on to achieve their short-term strategic goals.

- Each value stream involves many departments, and therefore much coordinated effort is required to accomplish strategic objectives.

- By focusing improvement efforts on the value streams that contribute most to the advancement of strategic initiatives, senior administrators provide direction and consolidate efforts.

CHAPTER 11

Map the Value Streams

See things as you would have them be instead of as they are.
—Robert Collier

Once the value streams are identified, their current and future states need to be mapped. The current-state map illustrates the value stream as it is presently operating. The future-state map portrays the desired state of the value stream. This desired or future state is based on strategic objectives and should not be confused with the ideal state. Although attainment of the ideal state is desirable, it is unrealistic and unlikely to happen, and one of the criteria of a SMART objective is that it be attainable.

After completing a multiday workshop on Lean concepts, including value stream mapping, the directors and/or managers of the departments involved in the value stream draw the maps. Value streams never should be drawn while sitting around a table and attempting to recall the steps involved. Ideally, the group should draw the map while following a patient or product through the identified value stream. However, if this approach would involve long wait times between steps (e.g., sitting with a patient in the waiting room), it would introduce waste. Instead, the group is advised to document the progress of one person through one step and then continue with another patient ready to start the next step.

In a value stream map, a process box represents a process in the value stream through which there is patient or product flow. If the flow is interrupted or stops, a new process box must be drawn. In a push system (in which upstream processes feed patients into downstream processes regardless of whether the downstream processes are ready to take the patients), interruptions involve wait times. The group must be sure to record these wait times between the process boxes (steps). Wait times are recorded separately from the times required to complete the process steps. The latter are recorded in the data boxes associated with the process boxes, and the former are recorded between the data boxes (see exhibits 11.1 and 11.2). When observation of wait times between steps is not practical because of their length, time stamps in the information system documenting progress through the steps in the value stream can be used to calculate wait times. Another option is to count the inventory (number of people in the waiting room), multiply that figure by the process cycle time, and then divide that number by the number of people performing the function. For example, if five people are waiting to register in the section of the value stream illustrated in Exhibit 11.1, the wait time for registration could be calculated as (5 patients × 16 minutes) ÷ 2 registrars = 40 minutes, which approximates the actual 42-minute wait time observed. Long wait times and impracticalities aside, all times (waiting, processing, transporting, and any other steps) should be obtained through observation whenever possible.

Exhibit 11.1 illustrates a process box for registration. The data box located below the process box contains the cycle time; takt time (the rate of customer demand), which is discussed later in this chapter; and the number of people performing the registration function. On the left side of the data box is the time the patient waited to be called for registration, and on the right side is the time the patient waited for the next process step to begin. This information is used to create a lead-time line, which is introduced later in the chapter.

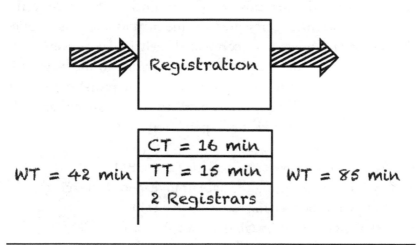

The value stream map is a high-level view of all processes that make up the value stream and depicts both physical flow (patient or product) and information flow (e.g., phone, fax, electronic) through the value stream. Because it is a high-level map, the amount of detail that would be documented for an individual process need not be included. This point is important to understand because the value stream map is possibly the most inappropriately used tool in Lean. Too often the value stream map is used during a kaizen event or for less significant improvement projects to illustrate flow through an individual process. The process map is the appropriate tool to use to define flow through an individual process (hence its name).

The following example illustrates the difference between a value stream map and a process map. Say a patient is sent from the emergency department (ED) to the diagnostic imaging department. At the value stream level, the reason a patient is going from the ED to diagnostic imaging—for example, for an MRI, a CT scan, a PET scan, an ultrasound, or a chest X-ray—is irrelevant. All that matters is that the patient is going to diagnostic imaging.

Exhibit 11.2 shows how this transfer would be illustrated on a value stream map. Notice that diagnostic imaging is not part of the ED process. Rather, this department provides a service to the ED and is therefore represented on the map as a supplier. Once the doctor and nurse have completed their initial assessment of the patient, the patient is physically transported to the diagnostic imaging department to undergo the diagnostic test(s) ordered by the ED physician. The wait time between ED assessment and ED diagnosis is the cumulative time spent on the following:

- Waiting for transport staff to arrive at the ED
- Physically transporting the patient to diagnostic imaging
- Waiting for the imaging service(s) to begin
- Performance of the imaging service(s)
- Waiting for transport staff to arrive at diagnostic imaging
- Physically transporting the patient back to the ED

Each process box illustrated on the value stream map is made up of one or more detailed processes. At the value stream level, all

Exhibit 11.2: Section of a Value Stream Map Depicting Patient Transport to and from Diagnostic Imaging

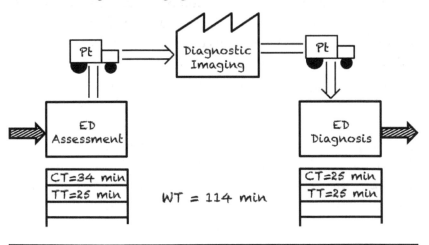

process boxes are viewed as adding value even though waste may be present in the integrated processes that make up a single process box. At this high level, "value added" simply means something is happening, not necessarily that it is being done efficiently.

Exhibit 11.3 illustrates a section of a process map for diagnostic imaging. In contrast to a value stream map, the level of detail mapped for this process is significant. This section of the process map identifies whether the diagnostic test requires use of a contrast agent and the test(s) to be performed. Each test involves a separate process (depicted in Exhibit 11.3 as "Next Process Step") that branches from this central process map section. This example includes five distinct branching processes (i.e., X-ray, ultrasound, CT scan, MRI, and PET scan).

Exhibit 11.3: Section of a Process Map for Diagnostic Imaging

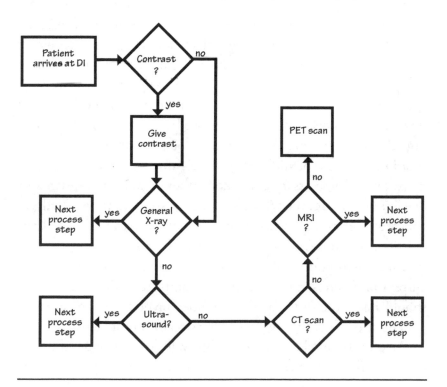

A value stream map is a pencil-and-paper tool. The use of Power-Point, Visio, or other expensive software applications, even those developed specifically for value stream mapping, wastes both time and effort. The purpose of creating a value stream map is not for it to be pleasing to the eye. Neat and orderly formatting often distracts from the real purpose of the map, which is to expose waste. Some argue that the value stream map should be computer generated for presentation purposes, but in a true Lean organization, this effort would be interpreted as waste and would therefore be inconsistent with any perceived benefits. The temptation to create computer-generated value stream and process maps is powerful, and people often try to justify the use of these software applications. No one wants to present a final product to superiors or peers that is less than perfect, but the waste generated by using such software is irrefutable. In their book *Lean Thinking*, James Womack and Daniel Jones (1996) describe the word *muda* (Japanese for "waste") as "an ugly word that sounds awful as it rolls off your tongue." If everyone in the organization internalizes these words and acknowledges that waste is ugly and repulsive, employees will develop an urgent need to eliminate all forms of it.

Symbols are used in value stream maps to illustrate flow through the value stream and to establish a common understanding of that flow. The symbols are not standardized and may vary from one organization to another, but they must be uniform within an organization. The use of different symbols on the same or different maps causes unnecessary confusion. If an organization designs its own set of symbols, the symbols should be simple and easy to draw. Fancy and elaborate symbols are difficult to recall and to draw, which again creates waste and slows down the mapping process. It is also important to label the different value stream maps as the current or future state. In short, the completed value stream map should make the order of the activities involved in processing a patient or product through the value stream comprehensible.

An often omitted component of the value stream map is the lead-time bar. The lead-time bar provides the data necessary to calculate process efficiency, a valuable piece of information. The sum of all the times (process times and wait times) indicated on the lead-time bar equals the total process lead-time. Similarly, the sum of all the process cycle times equals the value-added time. The value-added time divided by the lead-time equals the process efficiency.

THE LEAD-TIME LINE

Exhibit 11.4 features a lead-time line for a section of a value stream map. For this section the lead time is 249 minutes (the sum of all the process times and wait times) and the value-added time is 53 minutes (the sum of the process cycle times). Hence the process efficiency is 53 minutes divided by 249 minutes, or 21.3 percent. Given that all the tasks associated with the process boxes are viewed at this high level as value added, this low level of efficiency may be shocking, but it is not uncommon.

THE CURRENT-STATE MAP

In healthcare, improvement efforts are commonly directed at an individual process or department. The value stream map makes

---

Exhibit 11.4: Section of a Value Stream Map and the Associated Lead-Time Line

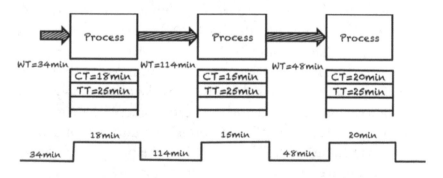

---

management and staff step back and view the entire value stream rather than strictly its discrete components. This atypical view is crucial to promoting systems thinking.

The current-state value stream map depicts the value stream as it presently operates. It also exposes waste and provides a baseline from which improvement can occur. Before putting pencil to paper, those in charge of drawing the map are advised to walk through the value stream to get a feel for how a patient or product currently moves through it, noting any obvious waste, problems, or obstructions to flow. To gain further insight, they should ask questions of staff members involved in the individual processes—for example:

- What do you see as the biggest obstruction to flow?
- Is this how the process runs on a typical day?
- Is this the normal staffing level and patient volume?
- What other tasks do you perform?

The basic process steps in the value stream sit in the center of the page, which leaves plenty of room above the process steps for suppliers and information flow and plenty of room below the process steps for data boxes and the lead-time bar. Again, the value stream map is a high-level view, so every possible scenario need not be captured. For ease of correction, maps should be drawn in pencil.

Finally, the use of proper, consistent symbols is essential. Exhibit 11.5 is a value stream map that includes incorrect symbols for a push system. Consequently, it does not depict patient or product flow or establish this value stream as a push system; instead it depicts manual information flow. This mistake is commonly made in healthcare, probably because healthcare workers are accustomed to drawing process maps. Exhibit 11.6 shows a section of a value stream map featuring the correct symbol (the push arrow). However, the absence of associated inventory (no inventory symbol) signifies a pull system, creating confusion for the person trying to interpret the map. Exhibit 11.7 features the proper symbols and illustrates the push process correctly.

A properly drawn value stream map is the starting point for the implementation plan. Therefore, the map must accurately represent the value stream and should include all pertinent information about the process steps in the value stream, such as cycle times, wait times, and changeover times.

The current-state map is sometimes considered inconsequential and only the future-state map is considered essential for success. Although a current-state value stream map is useless without

Exhibit 11.5: Example of a Section of a Value Stream Map Featuring Incorrect Symbols

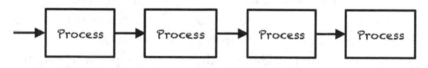

Exhibit 11.6: Example of a Section of a Value Stream Map Missing Symbols

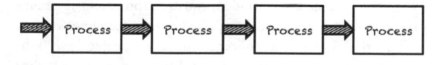

Exhibit 11.7: Example of a Section of a Value Stream Map Featuring Correct Symbols

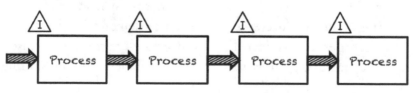

a future-state map, a properly drawn current-state map is critical to creating the value stream work plan. A lackluster approach to drawing the current-state value stream map will produce a faulty work plan and could jeopardize efforts to achieve the future state.

THE FUTURE-STATE MAP

The aim of your first implementation should not be to create an ideal future state. The future-state value stream map should be realistic, achievable before the start of the next fiscal year, and aligned with senior administrators' desired outcomes. Through continuous improvement, each value stream will be revisited, providing additional opportunities for improvement in the future. The future-state map can be designed by copying the current-state map and modifying it to reflect desired outcomes. It is advisable to draw the modifications in a different color so they stand out.

The goal of the future-state value stream map is to create flow through the value stream, so bottlenecks and other sources of waste need to be identified and eliminated. *Flow* means providing only what is needed to fulfill customer demand. The rate of customer demand, called *takt time*, is calculated by dividing available time by customer demand. The quotient equals the processing time allocated to provide a service to one patient or to process one product.

Takt time is a simple concept, but many people have difficulty calculating and understanding it for two reasons. First, they complicate the calculation with irrelevant information. Only two factors influence takt time: available time and customer demand. Available time and customer demand have an inverse relationship. If available time increases, takt time increases; if available time decreases, takt time decreases. If customer demand increases, takt time decreases; if customer demand decreases, takt time increases. All other factors, such as the number of patient rooms, staffing levels, equipment availability, bed status, and turnaround time for test results, are immaterial to takt time.

Second, people confuse takt time with cycle time (the actual time required to provide a service to one patient or to process one product). To better understand the difference between them, consider the following scenario. A service is provided during one eight-hour shift. It takes five minutes to provide the service, and the hospital has to process 100 patients per day (shift). The cycle time—the time required to provide the service to one patient—is five minutes. The takt time is calculated by dividing available time [(8 hours/shift × 60 minutes/hour = 480 minutes) – (2 breaks/day × 15 minutes/break = 30 minutes) = 450 minutes] by customer demand, which is 100 patients per shift. The quotient, 4.5 minutes, is the time allocated to provide the service to one patient. In this example, it takes 5 minutes to provide the service (cycle time) but 4.5 minutes are allocated to provide the service (takt time), so 100 patients cannot be processed in an eight-hour shift.

Once takt time has been calculated for the value stream, opportunities to meet takt time and create flow can be identified and highlighted on the future-state value stream map.

The future-state map provides an unambiguous picture of how the patient or product needs to flow through the value stream. The current- and future-state value stream maps provide the origin and the destination for the improvement initiative. Once these maps are in place, the only activities left to do are to create a plan for realizing the future state and begin the journey. These subjects are discussed in the following chapters.

SUMMARY: Map the Value Streams

- The current-state value stream map illustrates the value stream as it presently operates. The future-state value stream map portrays the desired state of the value stream.

- The directors and/or managers of the departments involved in the value stream draw the value stream maps.

- Because the value stream map is a high-level view of a value stream, the amount of detail that would be documented on a process-level map need not be included.

- The current- and future-state maps provide the starting point and the destination for the improvement initiative.

CHAPTER 12

Create the Value Stream Work Plan

He who fails to plan is planning to fail.

—Winston Churchill

How do you eat an elephant? The answer is "one bite at a time." This riddle refers to the best method for tackling big projects and is sound advice we have all heard in one form or another. Big projects are less daunting when they are broken down into smaller, more manageable tasks. The value stream work plan serves this purpose. The future-state value stream map identifies a destination, but without a plan for achieving the future state, the map has no value.

LOOPS

Division of the future-state value stream map into related functions is the first step in creating the value stream work plan. These divisions are called *loops*, and each loop is composed of interconnected flows. For example, inpatient admission from the emergency department (ED) is a complex value stream involving several departments and many functions. The first three processes that occur in this value stream are patient presentation, registration, and triage. These processes constitute a loop of interconnected flows. Assessment of the patient, diagnostic testing, and diagnosis might be the second loop of interconnected flows. Admission, bed assignment, and reporting might be the third loop, and so on.

The next step is to identify the improvements to be made in each loop. For example, the following objectives might be identified for the presentation/registration/triage loop:

- **Establishing continuous one-piece flow through the loop**: In one-piece flow, patients or products are processed one at a time, whereas in a batch-and-queue system, patients or products are processed in groups (i.e., batches).
- **Developing a pull system to enhance patient flow**: In a push system, upstream processes feed downstream processes regardless of whether the downstream processes are ready to accept patients. If the downstream processes are not ready, bottlenecks are created because the downstream processes are not processing patients as quickly as the patients are moving through upstream processes. As a result, patients must wait. This buildup of patients is "inventory" (equivalent to excess products in a warehouse that are "waiting" to be sold). Conversely, in a pull system, upstream processes feed downstream processes when the downstream processes are ready to accept patients, so patients do not have to wait (i.e., inventory does not build up). For example, instead of having 12 surgery patients all come to the hospital at 7 a.m. to register (regardless of their scheduled surgery time) and "pushing" them through to pre-op, which can accept only 3 patients at a time, patients could be told to arrive 45 minutes before their scheduled surgery time, and pre-op would be ready for them when they are done registering and thus would "pull" the patients from registration.
- **Reducing cycle times so they match takt times**: As discussed in Chapter 11, flow is created through the value stream when cycle times are the same as takt times.

- **Establishing kanbans in triage for necessary supplies**: A *kanban* (Japanese for "signal board") is a Lean tool used in pull systems. Kanbans are typically used to signal the need to replenish supplies, but a downstream process might use a kanban to signal an upstream process that it is ready for the next patient.

Some improvement efforts may be beneficial or necessary but not associated with a specific loop. For example, between triage and assessment of the patient, a room must be cleaned and prepared. If the team discovers that the time to change over a room is too long and is obstructing patient flow, the team can add a kaizen lightning burst to the future-state map, as illustrated in Exhibit 12.1. The kaizen lightning burst identifies the recommended action, in this case a changeover analysis.

VALUE STREAM WORK PLAN

After identifying the loops in the value stream and establishing improvement objectives for each, the team can develop the value stream work plan. The value stream work plan consists of the tasks that must be accomplished to create the desired future state in each loop of the value stream. Teams often have difficulty choosing a starting point for the plan. Among the several schools of thought

Exhibit 12.1: Section of a Value Stream Map Illustrating Loops and Kaizen Lightning Burst

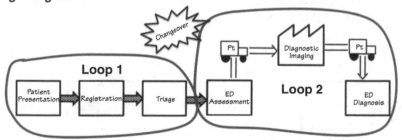

on this subject, the most commonly suggested starting points are the area with the greatest potential for success, the area in which implementation would be easiest, the biggest problem area, and the part of the process best understood by staff.

The ideal place to start, however, is at the end of the value stream. If the value stream work plan is initiated at the beginning or at any point other than the end of the value stream, the benefits achieved from an improvement event will likely be negated by the waste and inefficiencies present in downstream processes. By starting at the end and moving upstream, the team can build on the success of the previous event it worked on because it will have addressed any downstream constraints.

This concept can be illustrated by applying it to the section of the value stream shown in exhibits 12.2 and 12.3. Exhibit 12.2 illustrates a section of a value stream and inventory being pushed from one process step to the next. As shown in Exhibit 12.3, attempts to establish flow (pull system) at the beginning of the value stream or midway through it will cause an even greater pileup of patients

Exhibit 12.2: Section of a Value Stream Map Showing Associated Inventory

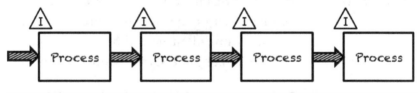

Exhibit 12.3: Section of a Value Stream Map Illustrating the Effect of Initiating the Value Stream Work Plan at the Beginning or in the Middle of the Value Stream

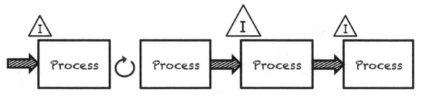

or products (inventory) at the next downstream process, as represented by the larger inventory symbol.

Conversely, if the pull system is created at the end of value stream between the third and fourth process steps, patients (inventory) cannot build up downstream because the downstream processes are pulling them from upstream processes. Exhibit 12.4 depicts a section of a value stream map that has been implemented beginning at the end of the value stream and moving upstream. As the work plan is implemented through the value stream, downstream processes do not hamper the successes of subsequent efforts.

Exhibit 12.5 illustrates the result of a properly implemented value stream work plan. When implementation is complete, the patient or product will flow from the first process down the value stream unobstructed.

This approach of starting at the end and working toward the beginning of the value stream does not exclude implementation

Exhibit 12.4: Section of a Value Stream Map Illustrating the Proper Method of Implementing the Value Stream Work Plan

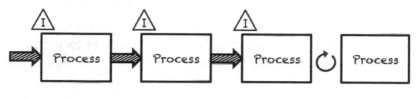

Exhibit 12.5: Section of a Value Stream Map Illustrating Unobstructed Flow Post-Implementation of the Entire Value Stream Work Plan

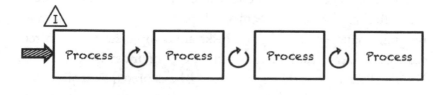

of less formal improvement efforts, such as the changeover analysis illustrated in Exhibit 12.1. Such small-scale efforts should be included in the value stream work plan but should be conducted at the departmental level. Obviously, the plan should identify any dependency the small-scale effort has on upstream improvement efforts.

Lean tools and concepts were developed to enhance flow. Some of the tools that directly affect flow include one-piece flow, pull systems, mixed model production, standard work in process, leveling, and physical layout. Other Lean tools and concepts target continuous improvement and waste elimination. In keeping with the goal of establishing flow, these latter tools and concepts indirectly affect flow. Standard work, kanbans, quick changeover, mistake proofing, and visual systems are included among these tools. Although the ultimate goal of any Lean initiative is to create flow through the entire value stream, this objective is unlikely to be achieved in the first iteration, given the variety and number of Lean tools. An attempt to optimally implement all these tools and concepts with a single value stream work plan can prove to be an extremely optimistic goal. The value stream will need to be revisited several times, each time improving flow and moving closer to its "ideal state." Therefore, it is imperative that the team stay focused and not deviate from its goal of achieving the defined future state of the value stream.

PROGRAM MANAGEMENT

Program management is an effort to organize and monitor implementation of the value stream work plan. A key responsibility of program managers is to ensure tasks are completed in the correct sequence. Some tasks included in the plan must be completed before other tasks can be initiated. These prerequisite tasks are called *predecessors*. Implementations of less formal improvement

Exhibit 12.6: Section of a Gantt Chart Used to Manage the Value Stream Work Plan

Value Stream Work Plan for: Value Stream 1

Task #	Task Description	P	Resource Names	Sept Week				Oct Week				Nov Week				Dec Week				Jan Week			
				1	2	3	4	1	2	3	4	1	2	3	4	1	2	3	4	1	2	3	4
1	Identified VS loop	2	Mary Jones Phil Brown																				
1A	The task or kaizen event scheduled	1B																					
1B	The task or kaizen event scheduled		Mary Jones Phil Brown Jane Doe																				
1C	The task or kaizen event scheduled																						
2	Identified VS loop		Larry Thomas Carol White																				
2A	The task or kaizen event scheduled		Donna Grey Janice Smith																				

efforts, such as the changeover analysis illustrated in Exhibit 12.1, are not usually dependent on the completion of other efforts and could be performed before, after, or at the same time as other tasks. Ideally, however, they should be scheduled and completed before upstream tasks are conducted so they can contribute to establishing flow. All elements—loops, objectives for each loop, nondependent tasks, predecessors, timelines, and necessary resources—should be defined in the value stream work plan.

A tool commonly used in program management to graph the value stream work plan and define order, duration, schedule, and progress is the Gantt chart. Each bar in the chart shows the time scheduled and the time actually taken to complete the task it represents. Exhibit 12.6 illustrates a portion of a Gantt chart. The bars representing the value stream loops span the entire length of time scheduled for completion of that loop. Each task involved in a loop is represented by a separate bar. The bars are filled in as time progresses and tasks are completed, thereby indicating progress relative to the schedule. The lines connecting tasks 1 and 2 and tasks 1A and

1B indicate that 1 and 1A are predecessors to 2 and 1B, respectively, and must be completed before tasks 2 and 1B can begin. The 2 and 1B in the P column also indicate this dependency. Necessary resources, responsible individuals, and other information can be added to the Gantt chart as necessary.

Microsoft Project is a useful tool for program management. It is less time consuming to generate and manage the value stream work plan in Microsoft Project than to create and update Gantt charts manually, but significant time must be devoted to learning and mastering this application. If program managers are already proficient at this software, it is beneficial to use because staff in different areas of the organization can access the Gantt chart for updates and status checks at the same time without having to schedule a meeting. Gantt charts should be displayed along with the continuous improvement status board and A3 reports in the responsible departments.

Proper planning is an essential step in any initiative. Creation of a detailed, unambiguous value stream work plan for achieving the future state is instrumental to changing and improving a hospital's care delivery system.

SUMMARY: Create the Value Stream Work Plan

- Big projects are less daunting when they are divided into smaller, more manageable tasks.

- Division of the future-state value stream map into related functions called loops is the first step in creating the value stream work plan.

- The value stream work plan should begin at the end of the value stream and progress toward the beginning.

- Program management is an effort to organize and monitor implementation of the value stream work plan.

CHAPTER 13

Strategy Deployment

Accountability for results rests at the very core of the continuous improvement movement.
    —Connors, Smith, and Hickman, in *The Oz Principle*

In many organizations, the strategic plan and the operating plan necessary to bring the strategic goals to fruition are developed in isolation. Often only a handful of key executives are privy to these plans, and they tend to communicate strategic objectives to staff improperly. Unless staff members are made aware of the hospital's vision, the plan for realizing that vision, and their role in achieving it, little progress will be made. Therefore, the next step in the Lean implementation model is to communicate the strategic plan to the staff, establish individual objectives, and make individuals accountable for accomplishing the strategic objectives in their areas of influence—in other words, to deploy the organization's strategy. Strategy deployment aligns the strategic initiative vertically and horizontally and ensures that the entire organization is focused on achieving the vital few objectives that will create success as opposed to the trivial many that will have everyone running off in different directions. This Pareto principle approach (i.e., 80 percent of the effects come from 20 percent of the causes) concentrates efforts on each year's strategic objectives and brings the organization significantly closer to its ultimate vision.

As illustrated in Exhibit 13.1, strategy deployment is critical to executing the strategic initiative successfully, but this step is often skipped because senior administration assumes that everyone has a clear understanding of what the organization is trying to accomplish. Senior leaders should keep in mind the adage "What's clear to you, is clear to you" and remember that what is obvious to them may not be obvious to staff.

When directors, managers, and staff members lack strategic direction, they naturally adopt a departmental focus. They believe that by focusing on their department's performance metrics they are exhibiting their department's value to the organization as well as their individual contributions. They work hard to meet budget requirements, reduce error rates, and minimize patient complaints—whatever is necessary to get the job done. To meet their departmental goals, they often resort to workarounds and stopgap measures, hide problems, and fail to report errors. They might even manipulate performance indicators. Consequently, the self-imposed goals and agendas of these departments often conflict with those of the organization. Consistent with a departmental

Exhibit 13.1: Strategic Planning and Implementation Process

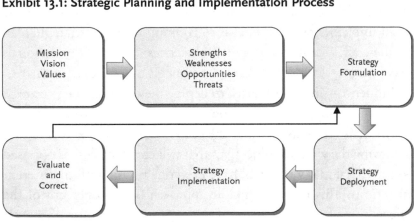

focus, the department's needs sometimes take priority over what is best for the organization or for patients. Because these departments consistently report good results, they are seldom identified as constraints to the delivery of patient care.

In reality, a departmental focus is extremely detrimental to the organization as a whole. To consistently produce desired results and be recognized as assets to the organization, departments may erect barriers to prevent other departments from influencing their performance, even when department interaction is in the best interest of the organization or patients. In so doing, they create silos. Silos inhibit patient and information flow through the value stream, breeding dissension and circumventing progress. Departmental silos compete for resources, attention, and positioning in the organization rather than encourage teamwork and focus on delivering the best possible care for their patients. When other departments attempt to breach these boundaries, turf wars erupt, reinforcing or even intensifying the silo mentality. Silos incite mistrust, blame, victimization, communication breakdowns, errors, inefficiencies, ineffectiveness, obstructions to flow, poor morale, and more. To create uniform, balanced flow and achieve the desired future state of the value stream, the organization must tear down these departmental boundaries. Strategy deployment is the first step to creating cross-departmental support of the Lean initiative.

STRATEGY DEPLOYMENT

The most effective method for communicating the strategic plan is to align the plan objectives horizontally and then cascade them vertically through the organization's hierarchy.

The strategy deployment hierarchy can best be explained using the organizational chart shown in Exhibit 13.2. The senior leadership team, which comprises the top two levels of the hierarchy (CEO, other chief officers, and vice presidents [VPs]), identifies the organization's areas of strategic focus and interrelated strategic objectives for the coming fiscal year. Subsequently, each VP/chief officer conducts a strategy deployment session with each director (the third level down the hierarchy) relevant to the VP's/chief officer's goals. Each director then conducts strategy deployment sessions with the department managers relevant to the director's goals.

Responsibility for the areas of strategic focus spans all major management disciplines. For example, quality objectives are not assigned solely to the chief nursing officer (CNO) and financial goals do not fall solely to the chief financial officer (CFO). The VPs/chief officers of all major management disciplines share responsibility for plan objectives and thereby establish horizontal alignment of the strategic initiative. By requiring that all departments in the value stream collaborate for the welfare of the patient and the enrichment of the care delivery process, the organization encourages a cooperative value stream focus rather than a defensive departmental focus.

For each area of strategic focus, specific annual goals are established to move the organization toward its principal strategic vision. Through horizontal and vertical dissemination and alignment of goals throughout the hospital's disciplines and management levels, staff members at every level of the organization can see how their efforts contribute to the betterment of the hospital. For example,

Exhibit 13.2: Strategy Deployment Hierarchy

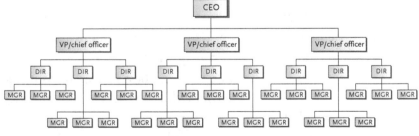

if employee satisfaction is an area of strategic focus, a goal for this area might be to achieve a nurse retention rate of 90 percent by the end of the fiscal year. This goal may have been established as a result of the following example scenario: During the strategy deployment session between the CEO, other chief officers, and VPs, the CNO presents data that indicate nurses decide within the first two weeks of employment whether they plan to stay with the hospital or seek employment elsewhere. In other words, nurses make this decision during their orientation period. The CNO feels that the existing orientation program is too short and inadequate. As a result, the VP of human resources is assigned the goal of revising the hospital's orientation program. To help the VP accomplish this goal, the CNO is assigned the task of identifying key weaknesses in the existing program and providing that information to the VP of human resources so he can make appropriate revisions. At subsequent strategy deployment sessions (between the chief officers, VPs, and directors), the CNO and VP of human resources assign goals to the director of quality improvement and the director of education services, respectively. Exhibit 13.3 illustrates the assignment of these goals.

Other members of the senior leadership team also share responsibility for the realization of this strategic objective. Most of the team's members have specific assignments that contribute to achieving the nurse retention goal. Some of these assignments are directly associated with the strategic objective, and others have more of a supporting function (e.g., the survey assignment in Exhibit 13.3 supports the revision of the orientation program). These goals cascade down through the organization to whatever level can best fulfill them. All levels of management can see how their goals for the year tie into the organization's strategic objectives.

An additional advantage of strategy deployment is the emotion generated when individuals see how their efforts benefit the organization. This emotion transcends the sense of accomplishment derived from goal achievement. When people feel they are instrumental to the organization's success, they develop a sense of

Exhibit 13.3: Example of Cascading Goals That Create Horizontal and Vertical Alignment of Strategic Objectives

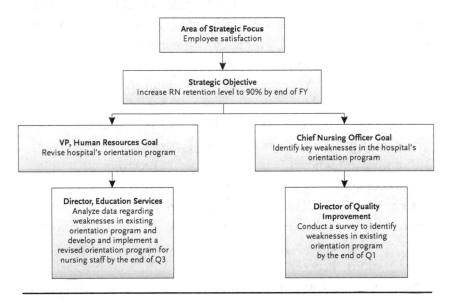

ownership and pride and act accordingly. Similarly, senior administrators recognize that staff members are the organization's most valuable assets, and their behavior reflects this realization. As discussed in previous chapters, this supporting element of Lean culture, respect for people, is possibly the most vital to a successful Lean transformation.

Strategy Deployment Sessions

The primary function of the strategy deployment session is to establish a method for deploying the organization's strategic plan. These sessions bring the team leader (e.g., VP) and his direct reports (e.g., directors) together so they can deliberate means of achieving the strategic goal assigned to the team leader. Direct reports are not told what to do; instead they help define what must be done. These sessions should encourage open discussion and be conducted off-site so they are not interrupted by the organization's daily activities.

Areas of strategic focus (ASFs) are an organization's principal outputs. The fundamental ASFs for hospitals and other healthcare organizations concern patients, care delivery, staff, and finances. Hence, a hospital might identify patient satisfaction, quality of care, staff relations, and financial stability as ASFs. Several objectives can be established for each ASF. For example, the quality of care ASF might have objectives related to reducing errors, enhancing services, reducing wait times, eliminating hospital-acquired infections, and reducing turnaround times. As the sessions cascade down the organizational hierarchy, the objectives become more specific. Each objective should have an associated metric (measure) defining the desired result. Upon completion of strategy deployment sessions, all participants should have a list of ASFs, objectives, and metrics for which they are accountable. The sum of everyone's efforts should be the realization of the organization's annual strategic goals.

The strategy deployment session is much more than a method for disseminating the organization's strategic plan. These sessions foster teamwork, build consensus for established goals, identify constraints that may be preventing team members from achieving their goals, explore the need for resources or other support, and establish accountability. These factors increase the probability of success exponentially. By assigning accountability, strategy deployment ties implementation of improvement projects to the responsible person's performance reviews. Without this accountability, daily duties can slow the momentum of improvement projects and eventually may even bring them to a halt.

As indicated in Chapter 10, the identified value streams should be the focus of the organization's large-scale improvement efforts, but those projects should not preclude other improvement efforts. Each department should have a set of additional goals linked to the strategic plan. These goals may or may not be associated with an identified value stream. If they are not associated with an identified value stream, these goals should be confined to the department's area of influence and should not interfere with efforts to achieve the desired future state of any of the identified value streams.

HOSHIN KANRI A3 MATRIX

One of the most common obstacles to successful strategy deployment is infrequent or no follow-up. Along with the continuous improvement status board, Gantt charts, and A3 reports, each department's ASFs, objectives, and metrics should be displayed on a visual management tool called a *hoshin kanri A3 matrix* so senior administrators can review them during their rounds. VPs and directors should formally review individual ASFs, objectives, and metrics with their direct reports at least quarterly.

The exact interpretation of the term *hoshin kanri* varies from one source to another, but it basically means a vector or a compass indicating the direction in which the organization should be moving. Similarly, the layout of the form itself varies, but the basic function of the layout is constant. A template hoshin kanri A3 matrix is provided in Exhibit 13.4.

The hoshin kanri A3 matrix is sometimes referred to as an X matrix because two intersecting diagonal lines divide the box at the center of the form into four triangles. The top and side triangles represent ASFs, objectives, and metrics. The bottom triangle represents results. Adjacent to the base of each triangle are cells in which information corresponding to the label can be entered.

Exhibit 13.5 shows the kinds of information recorded on the matrix. ASFs are directly linked to the strategic plan. The objectives and metrics are assigned to individual team members. The metrics cells are divided to display each metric and current performance relative to each metric goal. The results section identifies the organization's objectives and includes cells for the baseline metric, the targeted measure or goal, and the present status.

Exhibit 13.4: Hoshin Kanri A3 Matrix

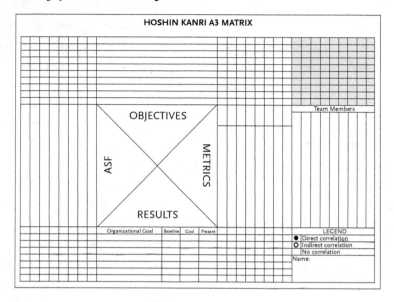

Exhibit 13.5: Instructions for Using a Hoshin Kanri A3 Matrix

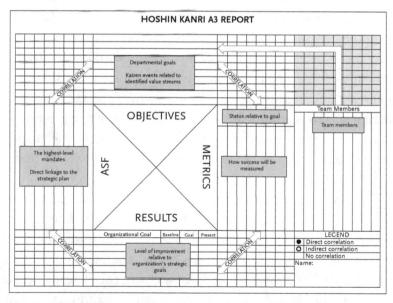

Exhibit 13.6 is an example of a partially completed hoshin kanri A3 matrix. As indicated at the lower right of the form, Mary Jones is accountable for this report. If Mary is a director or manager, her ASFs, objectives, and metrics are her department's ASFs, objectives, and metrics. Therefore, her completed matrix should be displayed along with the department's status board and its other A3 reports. The hoshin kanri A3 matrix should be updated whenever a status change occurs. Any updates (e.g., number of central line infections) or changes (e.g., reallocation of resources) should be identified in the quarterly hoshin kanri reviews.

The first part of the matrix to be filled in is the ASF section. In Exhibit 13.6, the organization's ASFs are patient satisfaction, quality of care, staff relations, and financial stability. Second, Mary's goals, established and agreed to during the strategy deployment session, are entered in the objectives section of the report. The two example objectives in Exhibit 13.6 are to implement a central-line checklist by the end of the first quarter (Q1) and to conduct a kaizen event for the pharmacy value stream loop 3. Next, the metrics associated with these two objectives are entered in the cells adjacent to the metrics section. In Exhibit 13.6, the metric associated with the implementation of the central-line checklist is zero central-line infections. The matrix indicates zero current central-line infections, but if any central line infections occur, the hoshin kanri A3 matrix should be updated to reflect the new status. The far right of the metrics section is completed with the names (not the job titles) of the team members assigned to the objectives. Finally, the hospital's measures along with the baseline metric, the targeted goal, and the current metric are entered in the results section.

The next step is to identify the correlation between ASFs and objectives, objectives and metrics, metrics and results, team members and objectives, and results and ASFs. The boxes formed by intersecting cells are used for this purpose. For example, the boxes in the upper-left corner of the form identify correlations between ASFs and objectives. As shown in the legend in Exhibit 13.6, shaded

Exhibit 13.6: Partially Completed Hoshin Kanri A3 Matrix

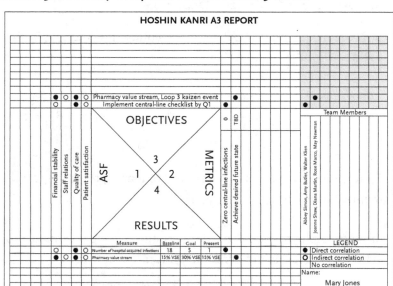

circles (●) are used to indicate direct correlations and open circles (○) are used to indicate indirect correlations. Blank boxes indicate no correlation. For example, Exhibit 13.6 indicates a direct correlation between the objective of implementing a central-line checklist by Q1 and the quality of care ASF; indirect correlations between this objective and the financial stability and patient satisfaction ASFs; and no correlation between this objective and the staff relations ASF.

Similarly, the correlations between objectives and metrics are identified. Each objective is associated with a metric. Several objectives may be associated with a single metric, and vice versa. Finally, the correlations between team members and objectives, between results and metrics, and between results and ASFs are identified.

SUMMARY: Strategy Deployment

- Strategy deployment is critical to executing the strategic initiative successfully.

- When directors, managers, and staff members lack strategic direction, their natural course of action is to adopt a departmental focus.

- Strategy deployment is the first step to tearing down departmental boundaries.

- Strategy deployment ties implementation of improvement projects to the responsible person's performance reviews.

- The hoshin kanri A3 matrix is an excellent tool for tracking progress and clearly assigns accountability for identified objectives.

Implement the Value Stream Work Plan

Success always comes when preparation meets opportunity.
—Henry Hartman

At this point, the time is ripe to implement Lean tools and principles at a multidisciplinary level. By now, the Lean culture should be ingrained in the organization. Staff should be familiar and comfortable with Lean tools and principles and should understand their role in achieving strategic initiatives. Departmental boundaries are beginning to crumble, individuals know what they are accountable for, and everyone is ready to start working to improve the identified value streams. Now is also the time to start conducting kaizen events.

All components of the culture-creating path are critical to success at this juncture. In the absence of a system-wide Lean culture, gains achieved through kaizen events will regress over time, so sufficient time must be allocated to cultural development prior to this point. Advancement from one phase of the implementation model to the next without providing adequate time for staff to become familiar with Lean tools and principles will not produce the desired outcome.

The definition of Lean—a system for the absolute elimination of waste—involves creating a care delivery system built around the patient and the patient's needs that operates as efficiently as possible.

Many components of Lean must function concurrently to produce this quality-driven system. The majority of the value stream work plan most likely will consist of a series of carefully planned and scheduled kaizen events. The kaizen event is the primary method for implementing Lean tools on a large scale throughout the organization and is the preferred approach to implementing change. Kaizen events should be conducted with the goal of developing standard work; creating user-friendliness; and establishing unobstructed throughput to improve efficiency, eliminate waste, and establish flow.

STANDARD WORK

In the absence of standard work, continuous improvement is not possible. One of the major problems in healthcare is the lack of consistency in the delivery of patient care. The methods doctors, nurses, technicians, and other staff members use to serve their patients vary—sometimes from one patient to the next, sometimes from one day to the next. The reasons for these variations in care delivery are too numerous to list. Hospitals that have implemented standard work have experienced significant benefits to the patient, the staff, and the organization. They save lives, save money, and improve productivity.

By establishing standard work, hospitals fulfill the criteria set forth by the Institute of Medicine (IOM). They provide care that is safe, effective, patient centered, timely, efficient, and equitable (IOM 2001). Unless care delivery is standardized, hospitals cannot guarantee that everyone receives care that meets all of these criteria. Standardized guidelines and best practices ensure earlier and consistent diagnosis and treatment of patients.

Every patient is different, and in some cases physicians may have to override standard work processes and make decisions they feel are in the best interests of the patient. The physician's liberty to take action he or she feels is necessary to treat a patient is a crucial component of any care delivery system, but this liberty should not be exploited as a premise to negate the need to establish standard work.

Standard work does not apply only to diagnosis and treatment. Standardization of testing, medication delivery, care transitions, administrative practices, and so forth is also necessary. These processes are laden with waste and inefficiencies that generate long wait times, errors, patient dissatisfaction, and unnecessary or duplicated efforts. Processes must be scrutinized closely to identify and eliminate wastes and inefficiencies, and standard work must be instituted to ensure the wastes and inefficiencies do not reappear.

Before waste can be eliminated, it must be identified. This task is more difficult than it sounds. Over the years staff have come to accept waste as inherent to their organization's processes and often view waste as necessary to care delivery. Waiting for information, making phone calls to obtain test results, clarifying orders, searching for medication or supplies—staff do not recognize these tasks as waste but as part of their jobs. Waste often masquerades as work, creating the false impression that busy equals productive. Staff cannot identify waste until they realize that the two (busy and productive) are not synonymous.

Even obvious waste often eludes staff's awareness. The following story is analogous to this phenomenon. After conducting a Lean healthcare workshop at a community hospital, I was invited to dinner with some of the hospital's senior leaders. On the ride back to the hospital, one of the vice presidents asked me if I had had any trouble finding the hospital. I told him that the town water tower outside the entrance to the hospital made locating the hospital relatively easy. The vice president replied, "What water tower?" Over years of working at the hospital, the vice president had become so accustomed to seeing the green tower looming over the hospital's entrance that it had blended into the landscape. Back at the hospital, we talked about our conversation in a wrap-up session, and several people in the group asked, "Is there really a water tower out there?" If we do not see a large, green tower emblazoned with bold black letters standing right in front of us every day, how readily will we identify the waste we have been accepting as part of a process for years or even decades?

To facilitate the identification of process waste, Taiichi Ohno, past executive vice president of Toyota, identified seven categories in which waste is prevalent (Ohno 1988):

- Delay
- Overprocessing
- Inventory
- Transport
- Motion
- Overproduction
- Defects

Delay, a predominant waste in healthcare, encompasses any time patients or staff wait. *Overprocessing* means doing more work than is necessary to complete a task or performing redundant tasks. *Inventory*, commonly considered a manufacturing waste, includes stockpiled goods or materials. Inventory is a greater problem in hospitals than it is in manufacturing because hospital inventory includes patients as well as healthcare supplies. Patients "pile up" in the ED waiting for a bed assignment, in pre-op waiting for surgery, or while waiting for discharge. One of the major problems with inventory is that it must be managed. In manufacturing, inventory management means cataloging, counting, rotating, and so forth. In healthcare it means all these tasks and much more. In hospitals inventory must be monitored, medicated, reevaluated, bathed, sent for tests, fed, and updated on their status, and staff often must deal with the family members of their inventory.

Transport includes any unnecessary transportation of people, equipment, specimens, and so on. *Motion* refers to excess movement, of which the most common manifestation in healthcare is searching. Staff members search for equipment, supplies, and medications, and they solicit assistance in their endeavor to locate missing items, compounding the amount of wasted effort. *Overproduction* occurs when patients, medications, specimens, and so forth are processed regardless of need, commonly referred to in Lean terminology as *pushing* (as opposed to *pulling*, which is processing as the need arises). Overproduction also creates waste in the form of inventory. The last of the seven wastes, *defects*, includes errors that occur regardless of whether they produce a defect. Staff who are familiar with (or better, who have memorized) the seven categories recognize and eliminate waste more easily than those who are not acquainted with them. Exhibit 14.1 provides examples of each type of waste in a healthcare setting.

Exhibit 14.1: Examples of the Seven Wastes in a Healthcare Setting

Waste	Examples
Delay	Waiting for bed assignments, waiting for treatment, waiting for diagnostic tests, waiting for supplies, waiting for approval, waiting for a doctor or nurse
Overprocessing	Excessive paperwork, redundant processes, unnecessary tests, using an IV when oral medication would suffice, multiple bed moves
Inventory	Specimens awaiting analysis, ED patients awaiting bed assignments, excess supplies kept on hand "just in case," dictation awaiting transcription
Transport	Transporting lab specimens, patients, medication, supplies
Motion	Searching for charts and supplies, delivering medications, traveling between wings to care for patients
Overproduction	Mixing drugs in anticipation of patient needs
Defects	Medication errors, wrong-site surgery, improper labeling of specimens, multiple sticks for blood draws, injury caused by restraints or lack of restraints

Even more complex than recognizing waste is the task of identifying specific process steps in which waste is present. Lean uses standard work forms to facilitate this task. The four main forms are the standard work sheet (used to identify waste in the form of excess motion), the time observation sheet (used to determine process cycle time and to identify waste in individual process tasks), the standard work combination sheet (provides a graphical representation of process cycle time relative to takt time), and the percent load chart (used to identify the distribution of work between people or shifts).

USER-FRIENDLINESS

The second element necessary to creating a solid foundation for the House of Lean is user-friendliness. User-friendliness is best described as providing for the staff member or patient what is needed, when it is needed, in the quantity needed, on time, every time, 24 hours/day, 7 days/week, 365 days/year. Such service may seem impossible to provide but it can and must be done. Staff cannot adhere to standard work if supplies are not readily available, if equipment is not in working order, if instructions are not clear, or if medications are not located where they are supposed to be. Several Lean tools help generate user-friendliness. The three most prolific are 5S, kanbans, and visual systems (discussed in Chapter 15).

UNOBSTRUCTED THROUGHPUT

The third element is unobstructed throughput, or flow. It is the ultimate goal of a Lean initiative and accordingly the most difficult to implement. Standard work, user-friendliness, and unobstructed throughput must be accomplished in concert; the absence of any one of these elements negates the benefits of the others.

A process flows only as quickly as its slowest task—i.e., constraint—progresses. Anyone who has experienced the exasperation of an overcrowded ED understands this principle. Regardless of how quickly a patient is triaged and assessed in the ED, how quickly laboratory and diagnostic imaging results are received, how quickly a bed is assigned, and how quickly transport can bring the patient to the unit, the patient will remain in the ED until the bed on the unit is empty, medications have been removed from the room, and the room has been thoroughly cleaned. In this case, room availability is the constraint. The level of collaboration necessary to move a patient from the ED to a unit is evident from this example. The ED, laboratory services, diagnostic imaging, the admitting office, the receiving unit, transport, environmental services, the pharmacy, case management, doctors, nurses, technologists, and other staff members must work together in the best interest of the patient. These departments and individuals have other duties as well. Pushing staff to work harder and faster will not eliminate constraints to flow. They already are stretched to the limit and doing their best to care for their patients. Only by standardizing processes and making them user-friendly can constraints be eliminated and flow established. The ultimate objective of the value stream work plan is to address the constraints within the value stream, thereby creating flow. Once a constraint to flow is eliminated, the next slowest process becomes the new constraint, and so on through the value stream.

Takt time, one-piece flow, mixed model production, standard work in process, kanbans, visual systems, quick changeover, and many other Lean tools must come together to create a pull system. The concept of "just in time" is key in creating pull. It means providing for the patient/customer what is needed, when it is needed, in the quantity needed, on time, every time it is needed. Maintaining a pull system in a healthcare environment has its share of trials and tribulations, but it will prove to be beneficial and will make schedule fluctuations and unexpected surges in demand more manageable. Another benefit of establishing a pull system is that it exposes the need for other process improvement initiatives. Using the surgical suite example, if the operating room is pulling from pre-op and a significant inventory of patients is still present in pre-op, this situation signals a need to create a pull system in upstream processes. Discovery of opportunities to improve is the basis of continuous improvement.

THE KAIZEN EVENT

The kaizen event, also called Lean event, kaizen blitz, or rapid improvement event, is best defined as the deployment of a team whose sole purpose is to implement Lean tools and concepts for the purpose of improving a process. These events are commonly scheduled for three to five consecutive days. The kaizen event is the primary method for implementing Lean tools and concepts in the value stream.

Kaizen events do not need to be scheduled for every loop of the future-state value stream map. Some initiatives may not require the intense focus and immediate action of a kaizen event; some may require collection and analysis of data and thus significantly more time to generate a successful conclusion. For example, an initiative to reduce room changeover time (the time needed to clean the room after a patient leaves and prepare it for the next patient) in the emergency department might require only a changeover analysis, which could be performed in half a day.

The value stream work plan identifies the value stream loops and any associated kaizen events or other improvement initiatives. Typically, a kaizen event entails five consecutive days of work by a dedicated team of six to eight individuals. By limiting the size of the team, the team leader is able to maintain control. Team members should have a thorough understanding of the process targeted for improvement, but inclusion of at least one team member who is not familiar with the process is advised. This person often identifies wasteful process steps and conditions that the other members of the team accept as circumstantial.

If someone cannot give a reasonable and legitimate explanation for any of the steps taken to complete a process, chances are the steps are unnecessary and wasteful. Moreover, a job that has been performed the same way for a decade or more is not guaranteed to be waste-free. Everyone in the organization needs to become keenly aware of how and why they conduct their duties. They must begin to look at processes objectively, through "new eyes." Instead of defending the process, they must be open to changing it.

The kaizen event follows the modified PDCA cycle illustrated in Exhibit 14.2. The cycle begins with documentation of reality and assessment of the current situation. In this first phase, the team maps the process, highlights constraints to flow, calculates takt time, and uses standard work forms to assess the current situation. By documenting reality, the team also establishes a baseline to which future improvements can be compared. In the second phase, the team uses the standard work forms completed in the first phase to identify specific process steps in which waste is present and to identify opportunities for improvement and plan countermeasures to address them.

Exhibit 14.2: Kaizen Event Cycle

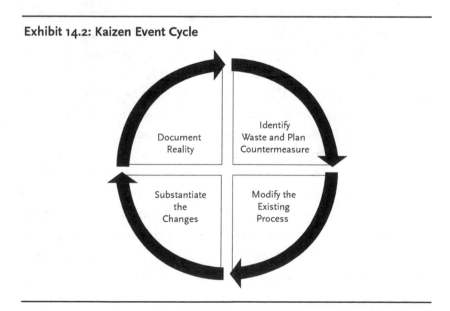

In the third phase, the countermeasures are implemented and the processes are modified accordingly. The team focuses on instituting single-piece flow, balancing the workload to promote flow, and eliminating constraints that inhibit flow. They may need to institute 5S, kanbans, and visual systems to establish uninterrupted flow. In addition, they may decide to employ poka-yoke (mistake proofing) in error-prone process steps to eliminate or reduce the likelihood of mistakes, and they might institute quick changeover methods to reduce the time required to switch from one task or patient to the next. The team leader monitors the team's progress during this phase and takes immediate action to alleviate any obstacles that hamper the team's ability to implement these modifications.

In the final phase, the team validates that the implemented modifications are producing the desired results. It may need to tweak the process and adjust for unforeseen circumstances. If further modification is necessary, the kaizen event cycle is revisited until the desired results are achieved. When the team is satisfied with the outcomes, it uses the standard work forms to quantify the results of the kaizen event and document the new reality.

Too often, events end with a presentation of the quantified results to the organization's senior leaders, and the kaizen event team members return to their daily routines. In so doing, the team neglects to adhere to a fundamental principle for creating a Lean organization: incorporation of new standard work. After a kaizen event, the team must establish the new standard work and disseminate it to employees involved in the process on all shifts to prevent them from resuming their jobs as they performed them before the event. New standard work is not established by drafting and distributing a document to the staff that demands they follow the new operating procedures. Instead, it involves explaining why the changes have been incorporated and providing any necessary training on the new procedures. All staff members assigned to the process on all shifts must participate in the training.

SUMMARY: Implement the Value Stream Work Plan

- Kaizen events should be conducted with the goal of developing standard work; creating user-friendliness; and establishing unobstructed throughput to improve efficiency, eliminate waste, and establish flow.

- Every Lean tool was developed to identify and eliminate process waste.

- The objective of the value stream work plan is to address the constraints in the value stream and thereby create flow.

CHAPTER 15

Heijunka and a Value Stream Focus

Flow principles can be applied to any activity and the consequences are always dramatic.

—James Womack and Daniel Jones

The system-creating path of the Lean implementation model concludes with the synthesis of heijunka and a value stream focus. Heijunka is the fourth element supporting the House of Lean depicted in Chapter 4 (Exhibit 4.2), and the value stream focus is the cross-member that ties all the supporting elements together. Heijunka would be impossible to achieve without a solid foundation of standard work, user-friendliness, and unobstructed throughput.

The goal of the system-creating path of the Lean implementation model is to establish flow through the entire process, or value stream. The delivery of care should be continuous from the time a patient enters the hospital to the time that patient leaves. Understanding the value stream, minimizing delays, improving process efficiency, eliminating obstacles, expediting changeovers, improving communication, and establishing more effective processes all contribute to the organization's ability to provide continuous delivery of care.

HEIJUNKA

Heijunka is the Japanese word for "leveling." The basic manufacturing concept behind heijunka is that the production of different models of a product can be uniformly spread out to meet customer demand. This idea can be difficult to transfer to healthcare, but for procedures that can be scheduled, such as surgery and diagnostic imaging, heijunka can be applied seamlessly.

Prior to 1914, Henry Ford's Model T was available in red, green, blue, or black. Between 1914 and 1925, Ford told the American public his Model T was available in any color, as long as the color was black. By mass-producing the car in a single color and incorporating a moving assembly line, Ford significantly reduced the cost of the vehicle and made it affordable for the average American.

The cost savings realized from manufacturing the Model T only in black had little to do with the cost of the paint. Rather, the savings resulted from not having to change from one color of paint to another. Furthermore, because Ford made only one model of car, the need to change over the assembly line to manufacture different models was not necessary. The price of the Model T dropped from a high of $950 to a low of $280. Using the consumer price index, in today's dollars this price reduction converts to approximately $14,000, from more than $20,000 to less than $6,000.

What does the story of the Model T have to do with healthcare? Patients do not have all the same symptoms and the same illnesses and cannot be cared for using the same treatments. But Ford does not manufacture only one model of car in only one color today, either. Auto manufacturers worldwide had to learn how to profitably manufacture different models of cars, trucks, SUVs, and crossovers in a variety of colors as well as offer a wide assortment of options. By applying heijunka—that is, leveling production by volume and product mix—they achieved their objective.

Heijunka involves seven components: just-in-time pull systems, one-piece flow, standard work in process, system replenishment, physical layout, mixed-model production, and quick changeover.

Just-in-Time Pull Systems

Just-in-time production (JIT) is a crucial component of heijunka. JIT is defined as providing what is necessary for the next process step, just in time (exactly when the need arises). This definition is based on the assumption that whatever is moving through the value stream—be it a patient, a specimen, a medication, or any other product—is provided in the quantity necessary to sustain flow, no more and no less. This idea is the essence of a pull system. As discussed in Chapter 12, a *pull system* is achieved when upstream processes supply downstream (subsequent) processes as the need arises. More succinctly, downstream processes "pull" from upstream processes, and no inventory builds up between process steps. In a *push system*, upstream processes supply downstream processes regardless of need or availability. For example, in a hospital push system, all patients scheduled for a particular test on a given day are told to arrive at 7:30 in the morning. They register and are sent to the waiting room, where they may sit for hours before they are called to undergo the test. In a hospital pull system, patient arrival is staggered so that patients arrive just in time to register and undergo their tests without delay.

One-Piece Flow

One-piece flow refers to having one patient or product processed sequentially to each process step without delay or interruption. For example, in Exhibit 15.1, at time equals five minutes, the patient at step 4 is discharged. The other three patients advance to the next step, and a new patient begins the process at step 1. At the end of every five-minute period thereafter, the same shift occurs. One-piece flow is straightforward in theory, but this example oversimplifies the task of implementing one-piece flow because the process is balanced (the cycle time for each step is five minutes).

Exhibit 15.1: Example of One-Piece Flow Through a Balanced Process

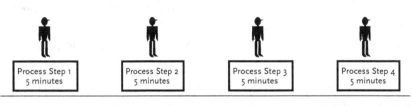

Standard Work in Process

Although no inventory is characteristic of pull systems, buildup of some inventory is unavoidable in certain cases. For example, if a process is not balanced, inventory is essential to establishing flow and balance. In such situations, standard work in process (SWIP)—that is, the minimum number of patients or products necessary to sustain flow—is maintained. The important word in this definition is *minimum*. Although SWIP is most often determined by trial and error, the following steps provide a starting point from which to calculate it.

The first step in establishing SWIP is to calculate the takt time and to determine the cycle times for each step in the process. Exhibit 15.2 illustrates an unbalanced four-step process. The cycle time for each step is displayed in the corresponding process box. For example, if the hospital determines it needs to process 225 patients through this process in one eight-hour shift, the takt time is calculated as follows:

60 minutes × 8 hours/shift = 480 minutes/shift.

The time for two 15-minute breaks is subtracted from the total time to determine the available time:

480 minutes/shift – (2 × 15-minute break) = 450 minutes/shift.

The available time is divided by the customer demand (number of patients) to determine the takt time:

Takt time = 450 minutes ÷ 225 patients = 2 minutes.

Exhibit 15.2: An Unbalanced Four-Step Process

| Process Step 1 2 minutes | Process Step 2 4 minutes | Process Step 3 6 minutes | Process Step 4 2 minutes |

Therefore, to meet customer demand, the hospital must process one patient every two minutes. Accordingly, the process steps illustrated in Exhibit 15.2 create bottlenecks at the four- and six-minute process steps (steps 2 and 3), causing patients to accumulate in the waiting rooms between steps 1 and 2 and between steps 2 and 3. As a result, delays occur at step 4, causing staff to wait for step 3 to be completed. SWIP eliminates or minimizes these bottlenecks and delays, but it does so at the cost of incorporating inventory into the process. Although SWIP creates inventory and delays in service—two categories of waste—an unbalanced process necessitates the use of SWIP to establish flow and meet takt time. The goal of using SWIP is to minimize the amount of inventory and the length of delays.

SWIP is determined as follows. First, the cycle time for each process step is divided by the takt time:

Step 1: 2 ÷ 2 = 1.
Step 2: 4 ÷ 2 = 2.
Step 3: 6 ÷ 2 = 3.
Step 4: 2 ÷ 2 = 1.

These values represent the number of patients being processed at each step. Exhibit 15.3 illustrates this distribution.

Exhibit 15.3: Distribution of Patients in an Unbalanced Four-Step Process

| Process Step 1 2 minutes | Process Step 2 4 minutes | Process Step 3 6 minutes | Process Step 4 2 minutes |

Second, the SWIP necessary between the steps to balance the process and establish flow is calculated by subtracting the number of patients in process at the current step from the number of patients in process at the next downstream step. However, if the number of patients being processed at the next downstream step is less than or equal to the number of patients being processed at the current step, SWIP is set to the number of patients being processed at the current step. In this example, SWIP is calculated as follows:

SWIP between process steps 1 and 2: 2 patients – 1 patient = 1 patient.
SWIP between process steps 2 and 3: 3 patients – 2 patients = 1 patient.

SWIP between process steps 3 and 4: 1 patient – 3 patients. As explained in the previous paragraph, more patients (three) are being processed at the current step than at the downstream step (just one), so SWIP is set to three patients.

Exhibit 15.4 illustrates SWIP at time zero. At this point the process is fully loaded. A disadvantage to using SWIP in healthcare is the need to reload the line every day; this factor is not present in most manufacturing processes. Daily reload reduces the available time and should be considered when calculating SWIP, especially for processes with longer cycle times.

Exhibit 15.4: An Unbalanced Four-Step Process Fully Loaded at Time Equals Zero Minutes

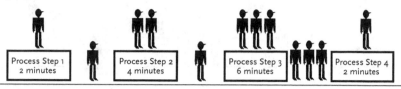

The use of SWIP enables this process to flow and meet the calculated takt time: Every two minutes, one patient completes the process and another patient starts the process. Exhibits 15.5 through 15.10 demonstrate the patient flow. At time equals two minutes, the patients at steps 1 and 4 are finished and advance. A new patient is brought into the process at step 1, and one of the three patients waiting between steps 3 and 4 moves to step 4. The distribution of SWIP at time equals two minutes is shown in Exhibit 15.5.

Exhibit 15.5: An Unbalanced Four-Step Process at Time Equals Two Minutes

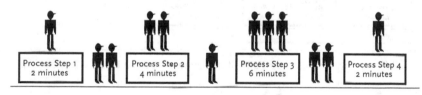

At time equals four minutes (two minutes later), another patient completes step 4 and a patient waiting between steps 3 and 4 advances to step 4. The patient at step 1 moves to the waiting area between steps 1 and 2, and another patient enters the process at step 1. At this time, the two patients at step 2 are finished (the cycle time for step 2 equals four minutes) and move to the waiting area between steps 2 and 3. Finally, the two patients waiting between steps 1 and 2 advance to step 2. The new distribution of patients is illustrated in Exhibit 15.6.

Exhibit 15.6: An Unbalanced Four-Step Process at Time Equals Four Minutes

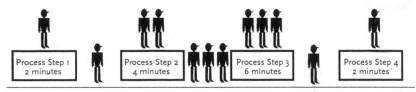

Every two minutes over the course of the day, patients are continually processed. Every two minutes, one patient completes step 4 and another patient begins step 1. Patients at steps 2 and 3 advance at multiples of four and six minutes, respectively. Exhibits 15.7, 15.8, 15.9, and 15.10 illustrate the distribution of inventory at time equals 6, 8, 10, and 12 minutes, respectively.

Exhibit 15.7: An Unbalanced Four-Step Process at Time Equals Six Minutes

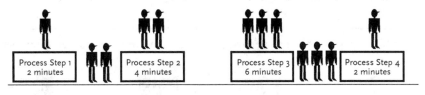

Exhibit 15.8: An Unbalanced Four-Step Process at Time Equals Eight Minutes

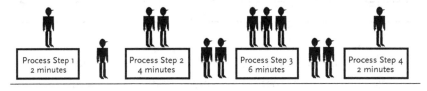

Exhibit 15.9: An Unbalanced Four-Step Process at Time Equals Ten Minutes

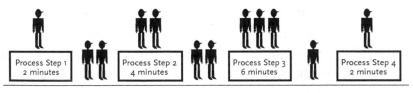

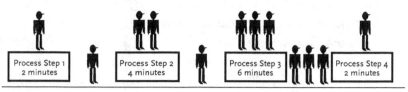

System Replenishment

The tool used in Lean to replenish systems or supplies is a signal called a *kanban*. The signal may be a card, a light, an empty bin, a color-coded square, or any other alerting device or method. A kanban may also be used to signal the need to advance a patient or product to the next downstream process step. The distance separating the upstream and downstream processes often dictates the type of kanban used. For adjacent processes, flags, lights, and similar visual devices work well. For processes separated by a substantial distance, a more elaborate kanban is usually necessary. Regardless of the form, use of a kanban reduces the time and effort involved in advancing patients or products.

Physical Layout

Excess motion is pervasive in hospitals. People in service jobs often are unaware of the effects of physical layout on the way they perform their duties. The physical layout of the work area may create barriers to flow; necessitate excess motion; increase errors; provoke redundancies; and waste time, effort, and money. Many architectural firms apply Lean principles to create innovative designs that help staff do their jobs more efficiently.

Unless a hospital is being built or renovated, work areas need to be reorganized to optimize physical layout. First, the work area should be clean, organized, and free of clutter. The Lean tool used for this purpose is 5S, which stands for sort, straighten, scrub, standardize, and sustain. Next, the distance between linked processes should be minimized. The standard work sheet, also known as a spaghetti chart, identifies excess motion necessitated by the physical layout of the process. Finally, to facilitate visibility and communication, hospitals should incorporate visual systems for nonverbal communication, including indicators, signals, controls, and guarantees. Bracelets for patients at risk of falling and NPO (nothing by mouth) stickers on patient charts are examples of visual indicators. Visual signals, such as lights and alarms, are used to attract attention. Visual controls limit behavior but do not prevent undesirable action. For example, a hazardous waste container limits improper disposal of hazardous waste but does not ensure proper disposal. Visual guarantees are mistake proof. For example, color-coded gas ports are visual indicators, but keyed gas ports are visual guarantees because they stop staff from connecting the patient to the wrong gas.

Caution should be exercised when changing the physical layout of a process. Facilities services staff should identify any conditions or hazards that may not be obvious. Preplanning with diagrams and schematics before moving equipment or rearranging large items is important to ensure the proposed layout will work as expected.

Mixed-Model Production

Mixed-model production is the practice of processing patients or products in a sequence that distributes the demand for downstream processes more evenly. Patterns in quantity and mix of services are identified, and a "smoother" schedule is created on the basis of these patterns. Consider a department that offers three services with the following cycle times: Service A = 20 minutes, service B = 30 minutes, and service C = 40 minutes. The department determines that daily customer demand requires providing service A nine times, service B six times, and service C three times. The resulting mixed-model schedule is shown in Exhibit 15.11. Mixed-model production is not always possible to implement but should be used whenever circumstances are conducive to it.

Exhibit 15.11: Mixed-Model Production Schedule

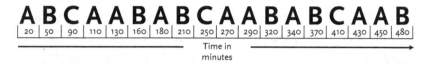

Quick Changeover

Inefficient changeover methods are costly and time-consuming. Recognizing this problem, Shigeo Shingo, a Japanese industrial engineer and an expert on the Toyota Production System, developed a method for reducing changeover times. In 1969, Toyota Motor Company challenged Shingo to reduce the setup time for a 1,000-ton press, which at the time took four hours to complete. Suddenly inspired, Shingo categorized the tasks required to complete the setup and converted or eliminated most of them. As a result, he reduced the setup time from four hours to three minutes (Shingo 1985). This feat convinced Shingo that any changeover could be accomplished in less than ten minutes. Accordingly, he called his new changeover system Single Minute Exchange of Die (SMED). *Single minute* refers to single-digit numbers of minutes—those less than ten.

Healthcare staff will never need to change over a 1,000-ton press, but they do need to change over operating rooms, patients' rooms, and exam rooms, and these changeovers cause delays and are constraints to flow. In addition, laboratory and diagnostic imaging equipment often needs to be changed over or set up. Shingo's changeover system also applies to these types of changeovers.

The SMED system divides changeover/setup time into two types: internal time and external time. *Internal time* includes tasks that can be performed only when the machine is not operating. They usually involve changing moving parts that could cause injury if the machine were running. In a healthcare environment, internal time translates to down time—for example, the time a patient room is vacant, the time post-surgery when a patient is moved from the operating room, or the time a diagnostic imaging machine is not operating. Internal time should be minimized, eliminated, or converted to external time, whenever possible. *External time* involves changeover operations that can be conducted while the machine is running. Changeover operations that could and should be conducted externally often are conducted internally. For example, equipment such as a scanner sits idle while doctors' orders are verified, patients' identities are ascertained, and test procedures are explained. These tasks could be performed while the machine is in use for another patient. Hospitals can reduce changeover time significantly—by 50 to 80 percent—simply by converting internal tasks to external tasks whenever possible.

In addition to converting internal times to external times and eliminating wasteful process steps, changeover tasks must be examined for efficiency. Tasks such as preparation, loading, and unloading; adjustments and alignments; and securing patients to exam tables before tests often can be performed more efficiently.

Heijunka is difficult to implement, but the rewards are tremendous. Work performed on the basis of takt time, implementation of one-piece flow, reduction of changeover times, creation of pull systems, development of mixed-model production schedules, and a focus on the value stream are essential to achieving flow and enhancing the care delivery system.

SUMMARY: Heijunka and a Value Stream Focus

- When implementing process improvements—the ultimate objective of which is to establish uninterrupted flow—hospitals should always consider heijunka.

- Heijunka involves seven components: just-in-time pull systems, one-piece flow, standard work in process, system replenishment, physical layout, mixed-model production, and quick changeover.

- Work performed on the basis of takt time, implementation of one-piece flow, reduction of changeover times, creation of pull systems, development of mixed-model production schedules, and a focus on the value stream are essential to achieving flow and enhancing the care delivery system.

CHAPTER 16

The Lean Enterprise

Accept the challenges so that you may feel the exhilaration of victory.
— General George S. Patton

The first effort to apply the tools and principles of the Toyota Production System outside the Toyota group occurred in 1987 at Danaher Corporation in Hartford, Connecticut (Womack 1998). Danaher Corporation's success with Lean was so impressive that by the early 1990s the US manufacturing industry had become a hotbed for Lean activity. Toyota laid out its philosophy for American companies to study and even copy. It entered into joint ventures, had books translated into English, allowed American manufacturers to visit its plants in Japan, and sent senseis (teachers) to the United States to instruct American manufacturers in Lean principles.

Results varied significantly from one manufacturing organization to the next. Some American manufacturers implemented Lean principles successfully; many more did not. The less-than-successful organizations embraced the revenue-generating, cost-cutting, problem-solving five-day kaizen event, believing they could implement select components of Lean and disregard the rest. Without a Lean culture and a system focus, they reduced Lean to a fire-fighting tool. To complicate matters further, many of the Lean facilitators quit their jobs and became consultants. With minimal experience in Lean implementation, these individuals conducted kaizen events in manufacturing companies coast to coast, forcing change on employees. They preached bottom-up implementation but practiced "do as I say" implementation. They told employees to work smarter but made them work harder. They talked about culture and systems but employed whatever tactics they deemed necessary to create change, but not necessarily change for the better. These consultants reprimanded workers, blamed management, pointed fingers at senior leaders, and advocated workforce reductions. They declared impressive results, but the results were short lived. Their implementation tactics soured employees to Lean, discouraged management, and confused senior leadership, and little improved.

In time, employees rejected the improvements and reverted to their old work habits. Managers allowed this retrograde to happen rather than attempt to enforce a methodology that they did not thoroughly understand. Fearing that these failures might affect their performance, they did not report the true status of their initiatives. To impart an illusion of success, they shifted attention to other areas or reported on the few processes that were working well. Senior leaders did not become aware of the widespread failure until several months later, after the consultants had moved on to other organizations.

Many of these consulting firms are infiltrating healthcare because of hospital leaders' yearning for quick fixes. Lean is relatively new to healthcare, yet many hospitals have already experienced the sting of improper implementation. Captivated by the results these consulting firms proclaim, hospital leaders surmise that by conducting more kaizen events, their organizations will achieve even greater results. Acting on this assumption, they hire these consultants. This approach poses several problems:

1. *It lacks strategic direction.* Without strategic direction, kaizen events fail to build on previous successes or advance the

organization toward its goal of becoming a Lean enterprise. This approach implies that the events are either financially motivated or a problem-solving tool. Kaizen events driven by either of these motivations generate impressive results, but the improvements are short lived because a Lean culture has not been established.

2. *The organization never learns.* The role of the consultant should be to transfer his knowledge and experience to staff to enable the hospital to continue its Lean journey independently. Rather than generate more work for himself, the consultant's job is to establish competency in the organization and render himself dispensable. Most consultants have no such intention. Their goal is to generate impressive results through one kaizen event after another, and they deprive the organization of the ability to sustain the Lean initiative on its own.

3. *It lacks enduring principles.* The kaizen event becomes the definition of Lean. Staff members and department heads come to dread the idea of having a kaizen event team swoop in and change their processes. They fear they will lose their jobs. Lean becomes an anxiety-inducing concept, and staff avoid Lean concepts rather than embrace them. They do not practice kaizen by questioning process operations in their daily activities. As a result, Lean never becomes "the way we do things around here."

4. *Gains backslide.* When the focus is on conducting as many kaizen events as possible, change is often imposed on staff members; they lack ownership. In time, they revert to comfortable and familiar routines, and the gains generated by the kaizen event are lost. Unfamiliar with Lean due to lack of training, staff members erroneously attribute the results of kaizen events to aggressive implementation rather than to the value and effectiveness of Lean tools and principles.

5. *It creates poor morale.* When staff are not consulted about proposed changes but instructed to follow newly established

standard work, modify the way they perform their duties, or discontinue certain activities, they become resentful and resist such directives. As a result, management must force change on the organization and attempt to drive people from their comfort zones. Both of these actions reduce morale.

Hospitals cannot afford to follow this quick-fix path to failure. If the Lean transformation is to be sustained, it cannot be consultant driven.

The Lean implementation model presented in this book is not a magic formula. It is a solution that only the courageous can initiate, only the vigilant can implement, and only the tenacious can sustain. For organizations that put forth the time, effort, and commitment required to create a Lean enterprise, the exhilaration of victory awaits.

SUMMARY: The Lean Enterprise

- The results of consultant-driven kaizen events are short lived and impart an illusion of success.

- Hospitals cannot afford to follow the quick-fix path to failure.

- The model for Lean transformation presented in this book is a solution only the courageous can initiate, only the vigilant can implement, and only the tenacious can sustain.

References

Agency for Healthcare Research and Quality (AHRQ). 2008. "New AHRQ Study Finds Surgical Errors Cost Nearly $1.5 Billion Annually." Press release, July 28. www.ahrq.gov/news/press/pr2008/surgerrpr.htm.

CBS News. 2007. "Eye to Eye: Donald Berwick." www.cbsnews.com/video/watch/?id=2440764n.

Centers for Disease Control and Prevention (CDC). 2000. "Monitoring Hospital-Acquired Infections to Promote Patient Safety—United States, 1990–1999." *MMWR Weekly* 49 (8): 149–53. www.cdc.gov/mmwr/preview/mmwrhtml/mm4908a1.htm.

Dictionary.com. 2011.

Encinosa, William E., and Fred J. Hellinger. 2008. "The Impact of Medical Errors on Ninety-Day Costs and Outcomes: An Examination of Surgical Patients." *Health Services Research* 43 (6): 2067–85.

Imai, Masaaki. 1986. *Kaizen: The Key to Japan's Competitive Success*. New York: McGraw-Hill/Irwin.

Industry Week/Manufacturing Performance Institute. 2007. *IW/ MPI Census of Manufacturers*. Cleveland, OH: IW/MPI.

Institute of Medicine (IOM). 2001. *Crossing the Quality Chasm: A New Health System for the 21st Century*. Washington, DC: National Academies Press.

————. 2000. *To Err Is Human: Building a Safer Health System*. Washington, DC: National Academies Press.

KLTV. 2006. "Airline Industry's Secret Safety Streak." www.kltv .com/global/story.asp?S=5114243.

Maltz, Maxwell. 1960. *Psycho-Cybernetics: A New Way to Get More Living Out of Life*. New York: Simon & Schuster.

Merry, Martin. 2003. "Healthcare's Need for Revolutionary Change." *ASQ Quality Progress* 36 (9): 31–35.

National Coalition on Health Care. 2010. "Thomson and Reuters Study Finds $3.6 Trillion Worth of Waste in Health Care System." http://nchc.org/facts-resources/thomson-and-reuters-study-finds-36-trillion-worth-waste-health-care-system.

————. 2009. "Containing Costs and Avoiding Tax Increases While Improving Quality: Affordable Coverage and High Value Care." White paper. http://nchc.org/blog/ nchc-white-paper.

National Public Radio. 2010. *All Things Considered: The End of the Line for GM–Toyota Joint Venture*. March 26. www.npr.org/ templates/transcript/transcript.php?storyId=125229157.

Ohno, Taiichi. 1988. *Toyota Production System: Beyond Large-Scale Production*. New York: Productivity Press.

Reid, Proctor P., W. Dale Compton, Jerome H. Grossman, and Gary Fanjiang, eds., for the Committee on Engineering and the Health Care System, Institute of Medicine, and National Academy of Engineering. 2005. *Building a Better Delivery System: A New Engineering/Health Care Partnership*. Executive Summary. Washington, DC: National Academies Press. http://books.nap.edu/openbook .php?isbn=030909643X&page=1.

Shingo, Shigeo. 1985. *A Revolution in Manufacturing: The SMED System*. New York: Productivity Press.

Shojania, Kaveh G., Bradford W. Duncan, Kathryn M. McDonald, et al., eds. 2001. *Making Health Care Safer: A Critical Analysis of Patient Safety Practices*. Evidence Report/Technology Assessment No. 43 (Prepared by the University of California at San Francisco-Stanford Evidence-based Practice Center under Contract No. 290-97-0013), AHRQ Publication No. 01-E058, Rockville, MD: Agency for Healthcare Research and Quality.

US Food and Drug Administration (FDA). 2009. "Medication Error Reports." www.fda.gov/Drugs/DrugSafety/ MedicationErrors/ucm080629.htm.

Vasishtha, Jagdish K. 2011. "Social Knowledge Workspace." In *Social Knowledge: Using Social Media to Know What You Know*, edited by John P. Girard and JoAnn L. Girard, 193–206. Hershey, PA: IGI Global.

White House Forum on Health Reform. 2009. Washington, DC, March 5. Report issued March 30. www.whitehouse .gov/assets/documents/White_House_Forum_on_Health_ Reform_Report.pdf.

Womack, James P. 2008. "The Toyota Concept of 'Respect for People.'" Cambridge, MA: Lean Enterprise Institute. www.reliableplant.com/Read/9818/toyota.

———. 1998. "The Lean Business System." Presentation at the Lean Enterprise Institute Summit, Hartford, CT, June.

Womack, James P., and Daniel T. Jones. 1996. *Lean Thinking: Banish Waste and Create Wealth in Your Corporation*. London: Simon & Schuster UK Ltd.

Womack, James P., Daniel T. Jones, and Daniel Roos. 1990. *The Machine That Changed the World*. New York: Rawson Associates.

Yasuda, Yuzo. 1991. *40 Years, 20 Million Ideas: The Toyota Suggestion System*. New York: Productivity Press.

Index

107–108; room changeover time in, 136

Empowerment, 20, 54, 63, 69–72, 72, 73

Error rate, 64

Errors. *See also* Medical errors: blame for, 65–66, 73; concealment of, 64; reporting of, 63–67; as wasteful process, 132, 133

Fear, 77, 157

Finance, strategic objectives for, 91

Financial focus, *versus* quality focus, 82–85

5 Whys method, of problem solving, 57

Flow, 104, 108, 112. *See also* Unobstructed throughput: constraints on, 135; as system-creating path goal, 141

Flow principles, 141

Focus: departmental, 25, 118–119; organizational, 48; strategic, 23, 24, 29, 48; value stream, synthesis with heijunka, 141–153

Food and Drug Administration (FDA), 79

Ford, Henry, 142

Fremont, California, General Motors plant in, 8–9

Frontline staff: problem-solving abilities of, 48–49; role in Lean implementation, 43–44, 50

Future-state value stream mapping/maps, 95, 104–105, 106; loops of, 107–109, 115, 130

Gantt charts, 113–114, 124

Gawande, Atul, 3

Genchi genbutsu, 48

General Motors (GM): government bailout of, 9; New United Motor Manufacturing Incorporated (NUMMI) joint venture of, 8–9, 20

Goals, of Lean, 112; for areas of strategic focus (AFSs), 120–121; departmental, 118; of kaizen events, 10, 134, 139; linked to strategic plans, 123–124

Guidance function training, 47, 49–50, 51

Habits, formation of, 17

Hartman, Henry, 129

Hazards, in work areas, 150

Health Services Research, 79

Healthcare costs, waste-related, 79–80

Healthcare delivery system, 80–81

Healthcare industry, craft model of, 78

Healthcare reform, 85; within individual hospitals, 3

Heijunka, 20, 36, 112, 141–153; definition of, 142; just-in-time pull systems component of, 143; mixed-model production component of, 150–151; one-piece flow component of, 143–144; quick changeover component of, 151–152; system replenishment component in, 149–150

Heywood, John, 63

Hirano, Hiroyuki, 55

Hiroshima, 68

Hoshin kanri A3 matrix, 124–127, 128

House of Lean, 36–37, 54, 63, 134, 141

Imai, Masaaki, 68–69

Implementation, of Lean, 5. *See also*
Departmental implementation:
"blitz" strategy for, 5–7; bottom-
up, 42, 156; consultant-driven, 12,
155–158; critical steps in, 5–6, 11,
13; culture-creating path of, 18–20,
21, 33–38, 63, 129; first attempts in,
155–156; improper, 5–8, 26–27, 28,
155–158; model of, 15–21; monetary
component of, 11; multidisciplinary, 129; nonmonetary component of, 11; organizational hierarchy
for, 42–44; strategic *versus* tactical
approaches to, 26–28; success rates
in, 7–8; system-creating path component of, 18, 19–20, 21, 77–94, 141

Implementation function training,
47, 50, 51

Improvement: as management function, 68–69; relationship to maintenance, 68–69, 72

Inconsistency, in patient care delivery,
130

Industry Week, 7–8

Industry Week/Manufacturing Performance Institute (IW/MPI) Census
of Manufacturers report, 7–8

Information management tasks, 88

Innovation, relationship to maintenance, 68–69

Input tasks, 90, 91

Institute for Healthcare Improvement
(IHI), 80

Institute of Medicine (IOM), 41–42,
130; *Crossing the Quality Chasm: A
New Health System for the 21st Century* report of, 85; *To Err Is Human*
report of, 41–42, 80

Internalization, of Lean concepts, 54,
58, 61, 62

Inventory, 108, 110–111; standard work
in progress-related, 145; unavoidable, 144; as wasteful process, 132,
133

Jidoka, 63-67. *See also* Errors; Standard work: as culture-creating path
component, 36, 54; definition of,
63–64; origin of, 63–64; synthesis
of, 20

Jones, Daniel, 88, 100, 141

Juran, Joseph, 55

Just-in-time (JIT) production, 143

Kaikaku, 68–69

Kaiser Foundation Health Plan, 80

Kaizen: as continuous incremental
improvement, 68–69; definition of,
20; responsibility for, 69

Kaizen events, 136–138; "blitz"
implementation strategy for, 5–7;
consultant-driven, 12, 155–158;
cycle of, 137–138; definition of, 136;
goals of, 10, 134, 139; improper use
of, 155–158; as Lean implementation focus, 20; as Lean initiative
platform, 37; managers' leadership of, 43; multidisciplinary, 53;
plan-do-check-act (PDCA) cycle
during, 56; pre-event training for,
6–7; process of, 136–138; purpose
of, 130; scheduling of, 26–29, 129,
136; standard work goal of, 134, 139;
strategically scheduled, 27–29; tactically scheduled, 26–27, 29; team

leaders of, 136, 138; team members in, 136–138; timing of, 129; unobstructed throughput goal of, 139; user-friendliness goal of, 134, 139; value map use during, 97; as value stream plan component, 130

Kaizen lightning bursts, 109

Kanbans, 109, 112, 134, 135; definition of, 149

Kano, Noriaki, 83

Kano Model, of customer satisfaction, 83–84

Kennedy, John F., 87

Key to Japan's Competitive Success (Imai), 68–69

Launch, of Lean initiative, 33–34; closing of, 44; improperly planned, 39–41; properly planned, 39–45

Lawrence, David, 80

Layers, 15–15

Leadership, organizational. *See also* Senior leadership teams: differentiated from management, 48; responsibility of, 25–26

Lead-time bars, 100–101

Lean: definition of, 77, 129; first realization regarding, 9–10, 12; quick-fix approach to, 156–158; second realization regarding, 10–11, 12; staff's negative attitudes toward, 7; staff's understanding of, 50, 61; standard work element of, 35, 36, 37, 38, 49, 50, 112, 130, 134; unobstructed throughput element of, 35, 36, 37, 38, 49, 50, 134–136, 139; user-friendliness element of, 35, 36, 37, 38, 49, 50, 134, 139

Lean events. *See* Kaizen events

Lean initiative: launch of, 33–34, 39–45; rumors about, 40

Lean organizational culture: culture-creating path in, 18–20, 21, 33–38, 63, 129; definition of, 9–10, 13; development of, 9–10, 12, 35–37; effect of departmental implementation on, 54

Lean Thinking (Womack and Jones), 88, 100

Lean tools, departmental applications of, 53–61

Lean transformation: patient care as incentive for, 41, 45; strategically directed action-based, 28, 29

Leveling. *See* Heijunka

Maintenance: as management function, 68; relationship to improvement, 68–69, 72

Management: differentiated from leadership, 48; improvement function of, 68–69; maintenance function of, 68

Medical errors, 41–42; failure to report, 66; as mortality cause, 80; potential, 67; reporting of, 66–67; surgery-related, 79

Medication errors, 79

Microsoft Project, 114

Middle management, role in Lean implementation, 43

Mission statements, development of, 23–24

Mistake proofing, 112

Mixed-model production, 112, 135, 150–151; definition of, 150

Model T, 142
Morale, 157–158
Motion, as wasteful process, 132–133, 149
Muda, 100

Nagasaki, 68
Natural selection, 81
Near misses, 67
Net income, 18
New United Motor Manufacturing Incorporated (NUMMI) joint venture, 8–9, 20
Nosocomial infections, 79
Nurses, orientation programs for, 121, 122

Objectives, strategic: achievement of, 23, 120–121; ambiguous, 92; communication of, to staff members, 117; correlation with areas of strategic focus (ASFs), 124, 125, 126–127; for healthcare quality, 90–91; horizontal and vertical alignment of, 122; identification of, 23; SMART, 91–92, 95
Ohno, Taiichi, 55, 132
One-piece flow, 112, 135, 138; case example of, 16–17; definition of, 143–144; of emergency department inpatient admissions, 108; as heijunka component, 143–144
Organizational culture change, culture-creating path in, 33–38
Organizational hierarchy: in Lean implementation, 42–44; in strategy deployment, 119–122

Output tasks, 90, 91
Overproduction, as wasteful process, 132, 133
Oz Principle, The (Connors, Smith, and Hickman), 117

Pareto principle, 117–118
Patient care: as incentive for Lean transformation, 41, 45; standard work approach to, 130–134
Patient registration, process box for, 96–97
Patient satisfaction, 83–84
Patient value streams, 88–89
Patton, George S., 155
PDCA (plan-do-check-act) cycle, 54, 55–56, 62
Percent load charts, 134
Pharmacy value streams, 91–92
Physical layout, 112
Physical transformation tasks, 88
Plan-do-check-act (PDCA) cycle, 54, 55–56, 62
Pneumonia, ventilator-acquired, 84–85
Predecessor tasks, 112–114
Preparation, relationship to success, 39, 129
Problem solving: A3 report use in, 56–58, 62, 124; cause-and-effect diagram use in, 57; of chronic problems, 3–5; continuous improvement status board use in, 58–60; 5 Whys method of, 57; frontline staff's skills in, 48–49; immediate, 54; as kaizen event focus, 26–27; by quality expert teams, 71; staff members' skills in, 48–50; staff's involvement in, 70–71; training in, 20

problem-solving skills of, 48–50; resistance to Lean, 41; role in Lean implementation, 42–44

Standard operating procedure. *See* Standard work

Standard work, 49, 50, 112, 130–134; absence of, 130; applications of, 131; as kaizen event goal, 139; as key element in Lean, 35, 36, 37, 38; new, dissemination of, 138

Standard work combination sheets, 134

Standard work in progress (SWIP), 112, 135; determination of, 145–149; disadvantages of, 146; as heijunka component, 144–149

Standard work sheets, 134, 150

Strategic approach, to Lean implementation, 27–29

Strategic direction: lack of, 118, 156–157; as support function responsibility, 47, 48

Strategic focus, 90. *See also* Areas of strategic focus (ASFs): goals related to, 122

Strategic plans: definition of, 23; deployment of. *See* Strategy deployment; formulation of, 23–24; strategic focus of, 90–91

Strategically directed action, 23–29

Strategy deployment, 48, 117–128; definition of, 117; follow-up to, 124–127, 128; hoshin kanri A3 matrix in, 124–127, 128; organizational hierarchy in, 119–122; Pareto principle approach to, 117–118; sessions in, 122–124, 123

Success, relationship to preparation, 129

Support, for Lean implementation, 24–26, 29

Support function training, 47, 48–49, 51

Surgery, errors during, 79

System, definition of, 77

System-creating path, of Lean implementation model, 18, 19–20, 21, 77–86; goal of, 141; interdependence with culture-creating path, 19; need for change element of, 79–81; obstacles to, 77; quality *versus* financial focus of, 82–85; value stream identification component of, 87–94

System replenishment, kanban use in, 149

Systems thinking, 11, 12, 13

Tactical approach, to Lean implementation, 26–27, 29

Takt time, 104–105, 135; calculation of, 137, 144–147; in standard work in progress, 144–147

Testing, standardization of, 131

Time observation sheets, 134

To Err Is Human (Institute of Medicine), 41–42, 80

Toyoda Automatic Loom Works, Ltd., 63–64

Toyoda, Sakichi, 63

Toyota Creative Idea Suggestion System, 72

Toyota Motor Company, 151

Toyota Motor Manufacturing Kentucky (TMMK), 9

Toyota, New United Motor Manufacturing Incorporated (NUMMI) joint venture of, 8–9, 20

Toyota Production System, 9, 64, 68, 155; andon cord system of, 69–70; respect for people component of, 69–70

Training: as cultural development element, 47–51; guidance function, 47, 49–50, 51; implementation function, 47, 50, 51; for kaizen events, 6–7; in Lean principles and tools, 34–35; in problem solving, 20; support function, 47, 48–49, 51

Transport, as wasteful process, 132, 133

Treatment, standardization of, 131

Triage, 109

Trust, between leaders and staff, 49

Understanding, of Lean, 50, 61

United Auto Workers Union, 8

Unobstructed throughput element, of Lean, 35, 36, 37, 38, 49, 50; as kaizen event goal, 139; as key element of Lean; as value stream plan implementation component, 134–136

Upper management, role in Lean implementation, 43

User-friendliness element, of Lean, 49, 50; definition of, 134; 5S tool for, 134, 138, 150; as kaizen event goal, 139; kanbans for, 134; as key element of Lean, 35, 36, 37, 38; visual systems for, 134

Value stream(s), 12. *See also* Current-state value streams; Future-state value streams: admission task component of, 88, 89; constraints to, 10–11; definition of, 10, 87–90; differentiated from process, 88; discharge task component of, 89; of emergency department inpatient admission, 107–108; focused effort in, 92–93, 94; identification of, 87–94; information management tasks component of, 88; input tasks component of, 90, 91; as Lean focus, 36; output tasks component of, 90, 91; patient value streams, 88–89; pharmacy value streams, 91–92; physical transformation tasks component of, 88; problem-solving tasks component of, 88; processing tasks component of, 90, 91; product value streams, 89–90; relationship to other improvement efforts, 123–124; service task component of, 89; support functions of, 10–11; takt time calculation for, 104–105

Value stream flow. *See* Flow

Value stream focus, synthesis with heijunka, 141–153

Value stream mapping/maps, 90, 95–106; computer-generated, 100; current-state, 95, 101–104, 105; for diagnostic imaging, 97–99; differentiated from process maps, 97–99, 106; future-state, 95, 107–109, 115; inappropriate use of, 97; lead-time bar component of, 100–101; as pencil-and-paper tool, 100; process boxes in, 96–97, 98–99; process of, 95; symbol use in, 100, 102–103

Value stream work plans, 107–115; components of, 109; creation of loop in, 107–109; downstream tasks

in, 108, 110, 111, 130; future-state
value stream loop divisions in, 107–
109, 115; Gantt chart use in, 113–114;
loops in, 136; predecessor tasks in,
112–114; program management of,
112–114, 115; properly implemented,
111; purpose of, 107; starting point
for, 109–112, 115; upstream tasks in,
108, 110, 111, 113

Value stream work plan implementation, 129–139; standard work component of, 130–134; unobstructed
throughput component of, 134–136

Values statements, development of,
23–24

Vice presidents, role in strategy
deployment, 119–120, 121, 122

Vision statements, development of,
23–24

Visual controls, 150

Visual guarantees, 150

Visual signals, 150

Visual systems, 112, 134, 135, 138, 150

Waste, in healthcare: as defects,
63–64; economic cost of, 79–80;

elimination of, 112; identification of, 47, 50, 51, 131–134, 137; in
process stream map creation, 100;
reports as, 56; standard work-based
reduction of, 131; in value stream
map creation, 100

Wasteful process steps, transfer of
responsibility for, 10–11

5 Whys method, of problem solving,
57

Womack, James, 88, 100, 141

Work areas, physical layout of,
149–150

Workarounds, 82–83, 118

Workshops, in Lean principles and
tools, 34–35, 49

Wright, Frank Lloyd, 15

X matrix. *See* Hoshin kanri A3 matrix

Zero error rate, 64

About the Author

Thomas G. Zidel is president of Lean Hospitals, LLC, a consulting, training, and facilitation company. With more than 25 years of experience implementing Lean and Six Sigma, he has guided many organizations on their Lean journey. A pioneer in Lean implementation in healthcare, Mr. Zidel has dedicated the last 11 years to working exclusively with healthcare organizations and has trained and mentored hundreds of healthcare professionals in the use of Lean and DMAIC methods and tools at leading US hospitals, including Yale New Haven Health System, The Johns Hopkins Hospital, and Aurora Health Care.

Mr. Zidel earned his bachelor of science in engineering from the University of Hartford and his master of business administration from Western New England College. He is the author of the best-selling book *A Lean Guide to Transforming Healthcare* and is a certified Six Sigma Master Black Belt.